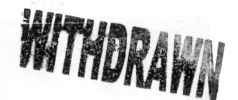

WA
900
BRI
REF
HJH P
(Bri)

All Change?

The Health Education Monitoring Survey one year on

The 1997 follow up to a survey of adults aged 16–74 in England carried out by Social Survey Division of ONS on behalf of the Health Education Authority

D1493839

Ann Bridgwood, Laura Rainford and Alison Walker
with
Mary Hickman and Antony Morgan

Edited by Tricia Dodd

OFFICE FOR
NATIONAL STATISTICS

HEALTH EDUCATION AUTHORITY

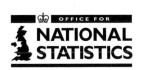
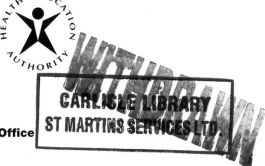
London: The Stationery Office

HEALTH EDUCATION MONITORING SURVEY (HEMS)

Other reports in this series:

Health in England 1995,
What people know, what people think, what people do (London: HMSO)

Health in England 1996,
What people know, what people think, what people do (London: The Stationery Office)

Contents

		Page
Project Team		v
Authors' acknowledgements		vii
Notes to tables		vi
Summary of main findings		**1**

Part A - Chapters 1 - 5

1	**Aims and background of the survey**	**3**
	1.1 Health promotion and models of behaviour change	3
	1.2 Design of the 1997 survey	4
	1.3 Focus of the 1997 report	4
	1.4 Changes between 1996 and 1997	5
	1.5 The future of HEMS	6

2	**Changes in smoking behaviour**	**8**
	2.1 Introduction	9
	2.2 Prevalence of cigarette smoking	9
	2.3 Changes in cigarette smoking status and consumption between 1996 and 1997	9
	2.4 Giving up smoking	10

3	**Changes in drinking and drug use**	**14**
	3.1 Drinking - Introduction and background	15
	3.2 Changes in alcohol consumption between 1996 and 1997	15
	3.3 Intentions and changes in alcohol consumption	16
	3.4 Perceived changes in drinking between 1996 and 1997	17
	3.5 Characteristics of respondents whose drinking has changed	17
	3.6 Drug use	19
	3.7 Changes in drug use in the last year	20

4	**Changes in physical activity**	**22**
	4.1 Introduction	23
	4.2 Participation in physical activity	23
	4.3 Change in participation at the individual level	24
	4.4 Intentions and change	25
	4.5 Perceived levels of change in activity	26
	4.6 Contributors to change	26
	4.7 Discussion	27

5	**Changes in diet and nutrition**	**31**
	5.1 Introduction and background	32
	5.2 Changes in eating habits	32
	5.3 Reasons for changing diet	35

All Change? The Health Education Monitoring Survey one year on

iii

Part B- Sexual behaviour and sun exposure tables   **62**

Part C - Reference section   **73**

Appendix A: **Sample design, response to the survey, weighting, characteristics of the**   **73**
              responding sample and sampling errors

A.1   Introduction   73
A.2   The sample design   73
A.3   Sampling individuals within households   74
A.4   The sample for the 1997 survey   74
A.5   Response to the survey   74
A.6   Non-response and weighting   75
A.7   The accuracy of the survey results   76

Appendix B: **Cognitive question-testing for the Health Education Monitoring Survey (HEMS)**   **92**

B.1   Background   92
B.2   Methodology   92
B.3   Cognitive question testing on self-reported stress   92
B.4   Whether respondents felt they were leading a healthy life   95
B.5   Physical activity   95
Annex B.1   HEMS questions and probe list   97
Annex B.2   Case studies   98

Appendix C: **Physical activity - Energy intensity categories and frequency measures for**   **99**
              different types of activity

C.1   The indicators of participation in physical activity   99
C.2   Energy intensity categories and frequency measures by activity type   99
C.3   Reference period   100
C.4   Modifications to the physical activity questions between 1995 and 1996   100
C.5   Measuring change   100

Appendix D: **Technical appendix**   **101**

Appendix E: **The questionnaire**   **102**

List of figures   125

List of tables   126

Project Team

Health Education Authority

Antony Morgan	**Head of Effectiveness and Monitoring Research**
Mary Hickman	**Senior Research Manager**
Karen Ford	**Research Manager**
Paige Sinkler	**Research Manager**

ONS

Joy Dobbs	**Research Director**
Ann Bridgwood	**Project Manager**
Nicola Iles	**Social Survey Officer**
Laura Rainford	**Social Survey Officer**
Michael Staley	**Computing Officer**
Peter Rowswell	**Assistant Computing Officer**
Jan Stern	**Field Officer**
Bhavna Amin	**Administrative Officer**
Nigel Hudson	**Administrative Officer**

Consultant

Alison Walker

Authors' acknowledgements

We would like to thank everybody who contributed to the Survey and the production of this report. We were supported by our specialist colleagues in ONS who carried out the sampling, fieldwork, computing and coding stages, and by our colleagues who helped us with the administrative duties. We would especially like to thank Nicola Iles, who was involved in the design of the Survey, and the production of the questionnaire. Thanks are due to the interviewers who showed commitment and enthusiasm throughout the Survey. We would also like to thank colleagues at the Health Education Authority, especially Paige Sinkler and Karen Ford, for their contribution to the Survey.

Most importantly, we would like to thank all those people who gave up their time to take part in this Survey, and showed such an interest in its aims.

Notes to tables

1. Where the base number is less than 30, numbers rather than percentages are shown in italics in square brackets.

2. The column percentages may add to 99% or 101% because of rounding.

3. A percentage may be quoted in the text for a single category that is identifiable in the tables only by summing two or more component percentages. In order to avoid rounding errors, particularly as the data were weighted, the percentage has been recalculated for the single category and may therefore differ by one percentage point from the sum of the percentages derived from the tables.

4. The following conventions have been used within tables:

    -   no observations (zero value)
    0   less than 0.5%
    [] numbers on a base of less than 30

5. Unless otherwise stated, changes and differences mentioned in the text have been found to be statistically significant at the 95% confidence level.

6. Values for means, medians, percentiles, standard errors (SE) and confidence intervals are shown to an appropriate number of decimal places.

7. Non-response and missing information: the information from an individual who co-operated in the survey may be incomplete, either because of a partial refusal or because the individual did not understand, did not know the answer or refused to answer a particular question.

    Respondents who did not co-operate at all are omitted from all analysis; those who did not co-operate with a particular section (e.g. the self-completion schedule) are omitted from the analysis of that section. The 'no answers' arising from the omission of particular items have been excluded from the base numbers shown in the tables and from the bases used in percentaging.

All Change? The Health Education Monitoring Survey one year on

Summary of main findings

Aims and background of the survey (Chapter 1)

The 1997 Health Education Monitoring Survey (HEMS) was a follow-up to the 1996 HEMS, where adults aged 16-74 in England were reinterviewed to see whether their health behaviour had changed in the intervening year. The survey was designed by the Health Education Authority (HEA), and developed jointly by the HEA and the Social Survey Division (SSD) of the Office for National Statistics (ONS) to contribute to the HEA's aim to:

- Provide sound, relevant information on needs and the effectiveness and efficiency of individual and community based health promotion activities.
- Inform policy locally, regionally and nationally.

Separate surveys were carried out in 1995 and in 1996, and the 1997 survey was designed specifically to look at changes in individual health behaviour by revisiting those interviewed on the 1996 survey.

Changes in smoking behaviour (Chapter 2)

Changes in cigarette smoking status and consumption between 1996 and 1997

- There was no significant difference in the proportion of respondents classified as current smokers in the two years. However 3% of men and 2% of women were classified as smokers in 1996, but not in 1997. The same proportion were classified as non-smokers in 1996, but as current smokers at the time of their second interview.

- Around three quarters of current smokers were smoking broadly the same number of cigarettes at the two interviews.

- About one in six current smokers were smoking five or fewer cigarettes in 1997 than they had in 1996. Just over one in ten smokers had increased their consumption by five or more cigarettes.

- Of current smokers who had increased their consumption by 10 or more cigarettes a day, around one half thought they were smoking the same number or fewer cigarettes than a year ago.

Giving up smoking

- For respondents who said in 1996 that they intended to stop smoking in the next six months, the odds of having tried to do so were five times as high as for those respondents who had said they were unlikely to give up.

- For respondents who said in 1996 that they had ever tried to stop smoking, the odds of trying to give up in the year before interview were almost four times as high as those for smokers who had never tried to give up.

Changes in drinking and drug use (Chapter 3)

Changes in alcohol consumption between 1996 and 1997

- Sixty-four per cent of women and 46% of men reported a weekly alcohol consumption in 1997 which was within three units of their reported weekly consumption in 1996.

- Respondents who reported drinking above moderate levels of consumption in 1996 were more likely than light to moderate drinkers to report a different level of consumption in 1997.

- Respondents aged 16-24 were most likely to report a weekly alcohol consumption in 1997 which differed by more than three units from that reported in 1996. Respondents in this age group were also more likely than older drinkers to perceive that they were drinking more than a year ago.

- People who thought they were drinking more than a year ago most frequently mentioned 'mixing with people who drink more' as the reason. Those who thought they were drinking less than a year ago most frequently cited 'change in work situation or social life'.

Drug use and changes in drug use

- Among respondents aged 16-54 who said in 1996 that they had used a drug in the past year, three quarters reported using a drug in the last 12 months in 1997. This compared with 4% of those who had not reported

All Change? The Health Education Monitoring Survey one year on

1

using a drug in 1996. Of those who had reported recent drug use in 1996, 54% were also 'current' drug users in 1997, having used a drug in the past month.

Changes in physical activity (Chapter 4)

Participation in physical activity

- In 1997, 26% of men and women were classified as sedentary. Thirty-nine percent of men and 30% of women were classified as achieving the internationally recommended level of at least moderate activity.

Change in participation at the individual level

- Forty-two percent of men and 45% of women had changed their activity group between 1996 and 1997 by more than one day a week. Men and women categorised as sedentary in 1996 were the most likely to have increased their activity.

- Most change was found among the youngest age-groups. More than half the youngest women had changed groups, with equal numbers increasing and decreasing their frequency of participation.

- Men and women who had 'left' the sedentary group since 1996 were most likely to have increased their home activities rather than any other activity; 60% of men and 53% of women who were sedentary in 1996 and active at least once a week in 1997 had increased their participation in home activities by at least one day a week.

Intentions and change

- Of those who said, in 1996, that they intended to take more exercise in the next month, only a fifth were more active than they had been at the time of the 1996 survey.

Contributors to change

- The odds of people increasing their participation in sports and exercise activities were five times as high for people aged 16-24 compared with those aged 65-75. Respondents' intentions (in 1996) to take more exercise and the time period in which they intended to do so were also significant factors in the increase in sports participation.

- Significant factors in increasing walking frequency or participation in home activities did not include the intention to take more exercise but did include the frequency of participation in 1996.

Changes in diet and nutrition (Chapter 5)

Changes in eating habits

- In 1997, 17% of men and 22% of women said that they had made a change to their diet in the last 12 months. Eating less fatty or fried food and snacks, and eating more fruit and vegetables were the most common dietary changes reported.

- Older people were less likely than younger people to have changed their diet.

Attitudes, intentions and changes to diets

- Respondents who said in 1996 that they wanted to change their diet in the next month or six months, were most likely to say in 1997 that their diet was different from a year ago.

- The most common reason for making a change was to lose or maintain weight.

2

All Change? The Health Education Monitoring Survey one year on

Part A - Chapters 1 – 5

Aims and background of the survey

The Health Education Authority's (HEA) research strategy, formally documented in 1997[1], aims to complement existing Department of Health and NHS Research and Development programmes and, wherever possible, to respond to NHS priorities. The overall aim of the HEA research strategy is to:

- Provide sound, relevant information on needs and the effectiveness and efficiency of individual and community based health promotion activities.
- Inform policy locally, regionally and nationally.

The Health Education Monitoring Survey (HEMS) makes an important contribution to the above aims at an individually based health promotion level. It was initially developed within the Government's public health strategy, The Health of the Nation (HON)[2]. Whilst HON acknowledged the impact of community level factors on the achievement of its health targets, health promotion's contribution was seen very much within the context of the knowledge, attitude and behaviour (KAB) paradigm[3]. Consequently the HEMS was set up to monitor the health-related knowledge, attitudes and behaviour of adults in England, using a series of health promotion indicators[4].

The survey was designed by the HEA in 1994, and has been developed jointly by the HEA and the Social Survey Division (SSD) of the Office for National Statistics (ONS), who have been commissioned by the HEA to carry out the HEMS surveys to date.

The HEMS surveyed adults aged 16-74 living in private households in both 1995 and 1996[5,6]. To date these surveys have performed two main functions within the HEA. The 1995 survey provided a baseline for monitoring knowledge, attitudes and behaviour, and the 1996 survey tested the validity of the measures used and provided the first set of trend data. The HEMS has proven to be a reliable source of information on health-related behaviour at a national level, presenting the opportunity to build up trend data across topic areas, including smoking, alcohol consumption, nutrition, behaviour in the sun, physical activity, sexual health and drugs.

Results from the 1996 survey confirmed that many of the indicators chosen for monitoring did not change appreciably over the two years. Therefore, whilst the HEA is committed to building up trend data over time and will continue to monitor health promotion's contribution to Government health goals, it was decided that this task could be carried out biannually. Therefore in 1997 the opportunity arose to consider other options. These included:

- selecting different indicators to be measured, for example those for mental health or accidents
- sampling a specific population group, for example different age groups or black and minority ethnic groups
- carrying out a follow-up survey of respondents from 1996

The decision to conduct a follow-up survey was made for two main reasons. First, collecting data in a cross-sectional survey provides a snapshot at one point in time. Whilst the samples in subsequent surveys will be comparable, analysis of change between cross-sectional surveys will not be as powerful as those between surveys looking at the same group of respondents over time. Secondly, looking at the same individuals at two time points has greater potential for uncovering the relationship between lifestyle and health. There is also greater scope for exploring more fully the relationship between intentions to change behaviour and actual behaviour change.

The aim of the follow-up survey was to compare data collected from the same group of respondents in 1996 and 1997. In particular it sought to:

- compare findings from the two surveys on health-related behaviour
- examine the relationship between intentions expressed in 1996 and changes in behaviour reported in 1997
- look at the relationship between life events and changed behaviour

Health promotion and models of behaviour change

The HEA's research strategy defined health promotion as the process of enabling individuals and communities to increase control over the determinants of health and disease and thereby to improve their health. The factors that influence and affect health do include aspects of individual behaviour and lifestyle. However, these factors also extend beyond the individual, to include the community, organisations, institutions and social structures. The wider context of the social, cultural, economic, political and physical environment in which people live has a major impact upon the experience of, and possibilities for, health and health promotion.

HEMS was initially developed to monitor targets set out in the Government's health strategy for England, *The Health of the*

All Change? The Health Education Monitoring Survey one year on

3

Nation, which was published in 1992. These targets were primarily to be met by encouraging changes in individual behaviour. For example, to achieve the main target of reducing the risk of lung cancer, coronary heart disease and stroke, risk factor targets aiming to reduce the number of people smoking were set. Similarly, reducing the incidence of skin cancer would involve reducing the number of people experiencing excessive exposure to the sun, and reducing the risk of HIV and other sexually transmitted infections would involve encouraging safer sexual practices.

The design and analysis of the HEMS surveys as a monitoring tool have been informed by two major influences: firstly by the HON targets; secondly, in order to understand health behaviour and its relationship to attitudes and knowledge, by two psychological models of behaviour change - the Theory of Planned Behaviour and the Stages of Change Model (**see boxes**).

These models represent complementary ways to understand health behaviour and its change. The Theory of Planned Behaviour attempts to delineate the factors which influence behaviour, whilst the Stages of Change Model provides an overview of the process of behaviour change itself. These models were used to inform all stages of the research, from the design of the questionnaires, such as the kinds and range of questions to ask, through the analyses, to the structure of the final report.

The 1997 survey therefore included questions that would make it possible to measure the association between attitudes and intentions expressed in 1996 and behaviour in 1997, as well as to measure respondents' movement through the different stages of change.

There are limitations to the application of psychological models to behaviour change, and these have been addressed in planning the 1998 HEMS (**see Section 1.5**).

Theory of Planned Behaviour
Ajzen's Theory of Planned Behaviour[7], an extension of the Theory of Reasoned Action[8] argues that a person's intention to perform a given behaviour is a function of three basic determinants: attitude towards the behaviour, subjective norms and perceived behavioural control. Each of these three constructs is held to be a function of beliefs: behavioural beliefs, normative beliefs and control beliefs, respectively. According to the model, it is necessary to change these underlying beliefs if behaviour is to change.

Stages of Change
The Stages of Change Model[9] has three dimensions: the stages of change through which people pass when changing their behaviour, the processes which they utilise to make changes, and the levels at which change occurs. The most recent version of the model postulates five stages of change:

- pre-contemplation
- contemplation
- preparation
- action
- maintenance

Successful change involves processing through the stages, from pre-contemplation to maintenance. Movement through the stages is a cyclical rather than a linear process, and relapse is the rule rather than the exception.

Design of the 1997 Survey

For the 1996 HEMS survey, a probability sample of addresses was selected from the Postcode Address file (PAF). Interviewers contacted each address and identified all residents aged 16-74. Adults within this age range were listed in order of age, eldest first, and one adult in the household was randomly selected to be interviewed.

At the end of the interview, respondents were asked whether they would be willing to participate in a follow-up interview one year later. Those who agreed were sent a 'keeping in touch exercise' (KITE) letter in January 1997, informing them of the intention to interview them again in the summer of 1997. As in previous years, an advance letter was also sent to all respondents prior to fieldwork, explaining the purpose of the follow-up survey. Full details of the 'keeping in touch' exercise are given in Appendix A.

In total, 4,323 respondents from the 1996 survey were contacted in 1997, of whom 80% (3,455) agreed to be interviewed. An additional one per cent (34) of eligible individuals were interviewed by proxy. Fieldwork was carried out in May and June 1997. More details of response and of attrition between the two waves of the survey are given in Appendix A.

Wherever possible, the same interviewers who carried out the 1996 interview were used to carry out the follow-up interview. If it was not possible for a HEMS interviewer to follow people who had moved, a telephone interview was carried out, which was of necessity shorter than the face-to-face interview. Respondents who had moved outside the United Kingdom were not followed up.

The 1997 interview lasted approximately one hour and the questionnaire was similar to that used in 1996. However, in order to exploit the follow-up nature of this survey, extra questions were added to explore changes in respondents' behaviour between the original and the follow-up interview. The full 1997 questionnaire can be found at Appendix E.

The interviews were carried out using lap-top computers. Respondents aged 16-55 were also asked to complete a self-completion module on drug use and sexual health. For the self-completion module, the interviewer handed the lap-top computer to the respondent, who keyed in the answers him or herself.

Focus of the 1997 report

Because of the follow-up nature of the survey, the main focus of this report is on the relationship between intentions to change health behaviours as expressed in 1996, and actual changes reported in 1997. However there is also some exploration of behaviours which occurred between the two surveys, which might have a bearing on changes reported in 1997; for example, respondents were asked about attempts made to give up smoking between the two surveys. As discussed above, respondents were also asked about important life events that may have occurred between the two surveys, and these data have been used to help understand more about changes in behaviour. These life events are described in more detail in Section 1.4 overleaf.

All Change? The Health Education Monitoring Survey one year on

It should be noted that, in general, unless otherwise specified, the age bands in this report refer to the age of the individual in 1996. Thus, for example, tables showing a comparison of those aged 16-24 in 1996 and 1997 will show the results for the same group of people, although in 1997 they will be aged 17-25.

To maintain the focus on longitudinal change, prevalence figures are given for each health behaviour, but trend data have not been reported in detail. At the end of each chapter the HEA has provided a short discussion of the implications of the findings and attempted to draw out the main conclusions for those working in health promotion.

Changes between 1996 and 1997

Changes that occurred between 1996 and 1997 could be related to changes in the circumstances of the people interviewed, or affected by events that had happened to those people in the intervening year. Table 1.1 shows the weighted[10] distributions for the socio-demographic characteristics for the sample as a whole in 1996 and 1997. It can be seen that, in general, the differences between the two years were relatively small. There were, however, quite substantial proportions of people who reported a major life event having occurred in the intervening year. (**Table 1.2**)

Experience of stressful life events has been shown to be associated with health-related behaviour; Melamed et al found an inverse association between stressful life events and participation in physical activity, and a linear relationship with smoking and alcohol consumption[11]. There is also a large body of literature showing that experience of stressful life events is associated with mental[12,13] and physical health[14]. Harris[14] notes that the link between stressful events and physical morbidity is not immediately evident; he argues that there may be intervening processes, such as the development of psychiatric symptoms, which could have physical effects. Alternatively, those experiencing stressful events may develop 'coping responses', including behavioural changes such as taking up smoking, which could have physical consequences.

HEMS respondents were shown a card listing a number of events, and asked whether they had experienced any of them in the 12 months between their two interviews. Whereas some previous surveys[15] have asked separately about adverse and positive events, HEMS included both 'positive' and 'negative' events on the card, as it was felt important to avoid introducing too 'negative' a note early on in the interview. A 12-month period was chosen because we were interested in finding out what had happened to respondents since their first interview. Although a shorter (for example, six months) period is often chosen for questions of this kind, there is evidence that reporting is adequate for a longer period when information is collected in an interview, rather than by using a self-completion checklist[16].
The events listed on the card were:

- Got married, started a new relationship
- Had a baby[17]
- Had a serious operation, illness or injury
- Close friend or relative had a serious illness or injury
- Death of close relative or friend
- Separation or break-up of a relationship
- Problems with neighbours
- Retired, started new job, changed jobs

- Lost your job/ partner lost job
- Problems at work
- Serious financial problems
- Personal experience of theft, mugging or other crime
- Family problems
- Other event[18]
- None of these

Women (75%) were more likely than men (69%), and younger people more likely than older respondents, to report that they had experienced at least one of the events on the card.

The most common event reported was the death of a close relative or friend; 24% of men and 23% of women had been bereaved in the last year. Women were twice as likely as men to mention family problems; 25% did so, compared with 12% of men. Just under one in five respondents said that a close friend or relative had had a serious illness, while changes associated with work such as retirement, changing jobs or starting a new job, and problems at work were reported by more than one in ten respondents. These results are very similar to those found by the Health and Lifestyles Survey (HALS2) follow-up survey; in that study, the most commonly reported event was a serious health problem of a family member or friend, followed by the death of a family member or the death of a close friend. (**Figure 1.1 and Table 1.2**)

Figure 1.1 Life events in the last 12 months by sex: adults aged 16-74 in 1996

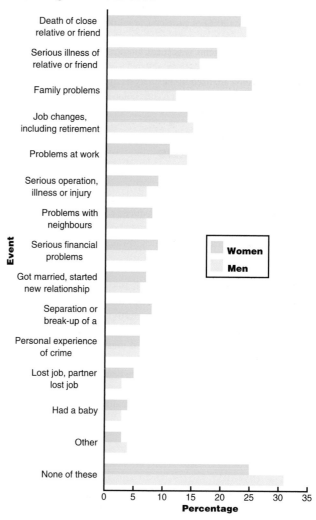

Base numbers are given in Table 1.2

Not surprisingly, as many of the events are associated with different stages in the life cycle, the likelihood of their being reported varied with age. Younger HEMS respondents were more likely than older ones to mention getting married or starting a new relationship; separation or the break-up of a relationship; having a baby; changes associated with work; financial problems and personal experience of crime. A higher proportion of the older age-groups reported a serious illness or operation, a serious illness of a family member or friend; or a bereavement. Problems with neighbours were most often mentioned by women aged 25-44; there was no clear association between age and the likelihood of reporting family problems.

The ONS Surveys of Psychiatric Morbidity[19] found that the strongest associations with life events were with economic activity status; unemployed respondents in that survey were five times as likely as those who were working full-time to have experienced two or more stressful events in the six months prior to interview. HEMS data were therefore analysed to see if there was a similar association and showed that 39% of men and 62% of women respondents unemployed in 1997 reported two or more events in the last year (**Table 1.3**).

To a large extent, this is a function of the events listed on the card, which include the respondent or their partner losing a job; a quarter of unemployed respondents said this had happened in the last year[20]. However, the unemployed were also more likely than other respondents to report family problems (30%), serious financial problems (22%), a marital separation or break-up of a relationship (19%). Not surprisingly, respondents who were working at the time of interview were most likely to mention changes at work (20%) or problems at work (18%). (**Table 1.4**: Data are shown for men and women together, as the number of unemployed respondents was small.)

These life events are used in the analysis of this report to help explain some of the change in health behaviour that occurred between 1996 and 1997.

The future of HEMS

Over the last five years the disease prevention approach of the Health of the Nation strategy has reduced some of the burden of disease. There have been significant changes in levels of knowledge about health, in attitudes towards health and in some health behaviours.

The two HEMS surveys carried out in 1995 and 1996 have supported the HEA's ability to monitor these changes in individual behaviour. The HEMS gives us a general picture of change over time and can highlight individual characteristics that have direct effects on this. However, it must be remembered that individual behaviour is only one of the determinants of health and there is an increasing need to develop a new set of indicators to reflect this. The Government's green paper 'Our Healthier Nation'[21] has highlighted the fact that health determinants need to

be considered within the wider social, cultural, economic, political and physical environment within which people live. Whilst it is still important for HEMS to collect information on knowledge, attitudes and behaviour to build up trend data, it will in future be necessary for the survey to consider other sorts of data, that could usefully be collected at national level, that reflect the wider context. HEMS 1998 has already begun to meet this challenge by collecting data, for example, on people's living conditions, their physical environment and the stress in their lives.

This shift also requires moving forward from the Theory of Planned Behaviour and Stages of Change models of health promotion discussed in Section 1.2. These models provide a useful framework for health promotion work, helping to explain some behaviours (particularly one-off behaviours such as attending health screening) and identify points of intervention, and offering insight into the factors which precipitate an attempt to change behaviour. However, they have been vulnerable to a number of criticisms. Importantly, these models view the individual as the unit of analysis or intervention. They ignore the connections between individuals, both the interpersonal and social relations in which they act and the broader social structures that govern social practice. The tendency to focus upon individual risk factors (e.g. smoking, diet etc.) fails to provide a more holistic interpretation[22] of health and well-being. Because these models are descriptive, there is no explanation of what causes motivation to change. The models can only suggest pre-requisites of change.

Therefore, in order to aid understanding of the wider context within which people adopt certain health-related behaviours, future HEMS surveys will also consider other models and frameworks.

Health and lifestyle surveys such as the HEMS provide an overall picture, which is important for planning at a national level. National organisations such as the HEA, need this type of information to inform their work. However, there needs to be a continual reviewing of the process, timing and suitability of the survey focus so that it can adapt to the changing environment of health promotion. For this reason the 1998 survey has not only broadened the focus of the questionnaire but also removed the upper age limit (formerly 74) from the sample. Thus the health knowledge, attitudes and behaviours of older respondents can be measured. Older respondents will also be asked an additional set of questions relevant to their age-group.

The broad topic base of the HEMS makes it a reliable monitoring tool for a variety of health promotion programmes at a national level, both inside and outside the HEA. Whilst HEMS collects a wealth of data, the published research report is only able to explore a small proportion of the information collected. It is therefore proposed that in the intervening years between biannual monitoring surveys, more detailed analyses will be undertaken on existing HEMS data sets, so that full advantage can be taken of this rich source of health-related information. HEMS data sets are also available for research projects through the Data Archive at the University of Essex[23].

Notes and references

1. Health Education Authority. Research for Health promotion: A research strategy for the HEA for England 1996-1999. A consultation document. Health Education Authority (February 1996).

2. Department of Health. *The Health of the Nation: a strategy for health in England.* HMSO (London 1992).

3. Buck D, Godfrey C and Morgan A. (1997) The contribution of health promotion to meeting health targets: questions of measurement, attribution and responsibility *Health Promotion International* Vol 12 No 3 pp 239-250.

4. Morgan A and Ford K. (1998) *A series of health promotion monitoring frameworks for use in demonstrating contributions to Health of the Nation targets.* HEA (London in press).

5. Bridgwood A, Malbon G, Lader D and Matheson J. (1996) *Health in England 1995: What people know, what people think, what people do.* HMSO (London 1996).

6. Hansbro J, Bridgwood A, Morgan A and Hickman M. *Health in England 1996: What people know, what people think, what people do.* TSO (London 1997).

7. Ajzen I. The Theory of Planned Behaviour *Organisational Behaviour and Human Decision Processes*, 1991, vol. 50, pp.179-211.

8. Fishbein M and Ajzen I. (1995) *Belief, attitudes, intentions and behaviour: an introduction to theory and research* Boston: Addison and Wesley.

9. Prochaska J O. (1994) Strong and weak principles for progressing from precontemplation to action on the basis of twelve behavioural problems *Health Psychology* vol. 13, pp 46-51.

10. For a description of the weighting process see Appendix A.

11. Melamed S et al. Negative association between reported life events and cardiovascular disease factors in employed men: the Cordis study, in *Journal of Psychosomatic Research,* (1997) vol. 43, 4, pp. 247-258.

12. Cohen L H. *Life events and psychological functioning.* Sage (London 1988).

13. Thoits P. Dimensions of life events that influence psychological distress: an evaluation and synthesis of the literature, in *Psychological stress: trends and research.* Academic Press (New York 1983).

14. Harris T O. Physical illness: an introduction, in Brown GW and Harris T O (Eds.) *Life events and illness.* Unwin Hyman (London 1989).

15. Whittington J E and Huppert F A. The impact of life events on well-being, in Cox B D, Huppert F A and Whichelow M J (Eds.) *The Health and Lifestyle Survey: seven years on.* Dartmouth (Aldershot 1993).

16. Funch D and Marshall J. Measuring life stress, in *Journal of Health and Social Behaviour*, (1984), vol. 25, pp. 453-464. Funch and Marshall also note that the frequency distribution of remembered events over time shows a fall-off of 5% a month for self-completion questionnaires, but 3% a month for interviews.

17. Both men and women were able to choose this option: equal proportions did so. When the 'other' answers were coded, 'got pregnant' was added to this option.

18. Respondents who reported an 'other' event were asked to say what it was. The answers were coded and three additional categories created (general worry or illness, housing problems or major DIY and important family event). However, because of the small number of respondents in each of these additional categories, they are not shown separately, but included in 'other' in the tables.

19. Meltzer H et al. *Economic activity and social functioning of adults with psychiatric disorders.* HMSO (London 1995).

20. Not all the life events were included in this analysis but only those where the individual had little or no control. These were:

    * Had a serious operation, illness or injury
    * Close friend or relative had a serious illness or injury
    * Death of close relative or friend
    * Separation or break-up of a relationship
    * Problems with neighbours
    * Retired, started new job, changed jobs
    * Lost your job/ partner lost job
    * Problems at work
    * Serious financial problems
    * Personal experience of theft, mugging or other crime
    * Family problems

21. Department of Health. *Our Healthier Nation: A contract for health.* TSO (London 1998).

22. Luepker R V et al. (1994) *Community education for cardiovascular disease prevention: risk factor changes in the Minnesota Health Program* American Journal of Public Health vol. 84: 1383-1393.

23. For further information, contact:

    Data Archive
    University of Essex
    Wivenhoe Park
    Colchester
    Essex
    CO4 3SQ

    Tel: 01206 872 001
    Fax: 01206 872 003

    e-mail: archive@essex.ac.uk

All Change? The Health Education Monitoring Survey one year on

7

Changes in smoking behaviour

Summary of main findings

- Three per cent of men and 2% of women were classified as smokers in 1996, but not in 1997. (Section 2.3).

- Three per cent of men and 2% of women were classified as non-smokers in 1996, but as current smokers at the time of their second interview. (Section 2.3).

- Seventy four per cent of smokers were smoking broadly the same number of cigarettes at the two interviews. (Section 2.3.1).

- About one in six smokers were smoking five or fewer cigarettes in 1997 than they had in 1996 while just over one in ten had increased their consumption by five or more cigarettes. (Section 2.3.1).

- A half (51%) of smokers who had increased their consumption by 10 or more a day, said they thought they were smoking the same number or fewer cigarettes than a year ago, while 36% of those who had decreased their consumption by 10 or more a day, said that they were smoking the same number or more. (Section 2.3.2).

- Smokers in 1996 who said that they had tried to give up smoking were more likely than smokers who had not tried to give up, to have tried again to give up smoking in the year between the two interviews. (Section 2.4.1).

- For respondents who said in 1996 that they intended to stop smoking in the next six months, the odds of trying to do so were five times as high as those for respondents who said they were unlikely to give up. (Section 2.4.1).

- For respondents who said in 1996 that they had ever tried to give up smoking, the odds of trying to give up in the year before interview were almost four times as high as those for smokers who had never tried to give up. (Section 2.4.1).

Introduction

Many of the psychological models of health behaviour change like those discussed in Chapter 1 were developed by using data from studies of smoking. This is understandable; smoking is widely recognised as a high risk[1] behaviour, with many adverse effects on health. On an individual level, it represents the greatest single self-imposed risk to health and, for smokers, stopping smoking would be more effective than any other change in behaviour in reducing the risk of premature mortality[2]. At a population level, the Health Education Authority has estimated that one in four deaths in the UK between the ages of 35 and 65 is smoking-related[3], while smoking is also associated with several types of morbidity, including lung cancer, peripheral vascular disease (P.V.D), and stroke[4]. The elimination of smoking would bring about considerable health gain at a societal level.

In this chapter, results from 1996 and 1997 HEMS are used to show how individual smoking behaviour changed between the two rounds of the survey, and to relate intentions to give up smoking expressed in 1996, with smoking behaviour in 1997. Before presenting this information about longitudinal change, the following section compares the overall prevalence of cigarette smoking in the two years.

Prevalence of cigarette smoking

HEMS measures cigarette smoking prevalence by using the same questions as those used on many other surveys such as the General Household Survey (GHS) and the Health Survey for England (HSE). Respondents are asked whether they have ever smoked; if they have, they are asked whether they smoke at all nowadays and, if so, how many cigarettes a day they smoke in the week and at weekends. It is likely that HEMS, like other surveys, understates cigarette consumption because respondents tend to round down to the nearest ten cigarettes. To a lesser extent, it is also likely to understate cigarette smoking prevalence.

This may be a particular problem for younger respondents, most of whom are interviewed in the family home. Those aged 16-17 complete the smoking and drinking sections of the interview themselves on the laptop, and interviewers are able to offer this option to older respondents if they feel that lack of privacy may jeopardise reporting. In 1997, 1% of respondents self-completed this part of the interview. The GHS uses a self-completion form for respondents aged 16-17, but a comparison of the 1992 GHS results with those from the regular ONS surveys of smoking among school children suggested that this age-group under-reported their smoking when interviewed in the family home[5].

Table 2.1 presents data on prevalence and consumption for HEMS respondents in 1996 and 1997. There was no significant difference in the proportion of respondents classified as current cigarette smokers, as ex-regular smokers and as never having smoked in these two years. In 1997, for example, 30% of men and 29% of women were classed as current cigarette smokers, 27% of men and 19% of women were ex-regular cigarette smokers, and 42% of men and 52% of women said they had never or had only occasionally smoked cigarettes. **(Table 2.1 and Figure 2.1)**

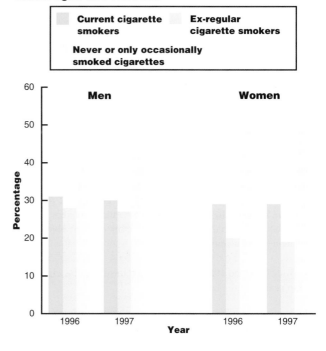

Figure 2.1 Cigarette smoking status in 1996 and 1997: adults aged 16-74 in 1996

As with other health-related behaviours discussed in the report, however, the apparent stability in cigarette smoking prevalence from year to year among HEMS respondents masks a degree of change at an individual level, as discussed in the following section.

Changes in cigarette smoking status and consumption between 1996 and 1997

Changes in smoking at the individual level are presented in Table 2.2 which shows cigarette smoking status in 1997 by smoking status in 1996. Those who said in 1996 that they had never or only occasionally smoked were most likely to be classified to the same group in 1997; 97% of men and 98% of women were in the same category in 1997, although a small proportion of this group had smoked at some time between the two interviews. Similarly, 89% of men and 90% of women who were ex-regular cigarette smokers in 1996 were classified in the same way at their second interview. The majority had not smoked between the two interviews, but a small proportion reported smoking at some time during the last year. More than 90% of 1996 smokers were also smoking cigarettes in 1997, although about a quarter had increased or reduced their daily consumption. **(Table 2.2)**

Interestingly, Table 2.2 shows that some of those who were classified as 'current cigarette smokers' in 1996 were allocated to the 'never or only occasionally smoked' group in 1997, including a small number of respondents who said at their first interview that they smoked 10-20 cigarettes per day. Respondents are classified as 'current smokers' by HEMS if they 'smoke cigarettes at all nowadays' and as ex-regular smokers if they say they have ever smoked cigarettes and, in answer to a question about how much they smoked, do not choose the option 'never smoked regularly'. Some of those who had stopped smoking between the two interviews and who told the interviewer in 1997 that they 'never smoked regularly' were evidently using a definition of 'regularly' which was based not on how much they smoked a day, but on some other factor such as how long they had smoked for. Alternatively, some of those who had given up smoking or who only smoke occasionally may think of themselves as not being or never having been a 'real' smoker, and this might cover those who think of themselves only as 'social smokers'.

The data suggest that the boundary between 'smokers' and 'non-smokers' is a fluid one and, as Marsh and Matheson[6] argued in 1983, that there is considerable traffic between these categories. It may be useful to think of a group of confirmed smokers who have never tried to give up smoking, a group which has never or only occasionally smoked cigarettes and a large group of people who move between the 'current' and 'ex-regular' smokers groups some of whom, when they quit, cease to think of themselves as ever having been a smoker.

Data from 1996 and 1997 were combined to summarise cigarette smoking status in the two years:

- 27% of men and 26% of women were smoking cigarettes at the time of both interviews
- 3% of men and 2% of women were cigarette smokers in 1996, but not in 1997
- 3% of men and 2% of women were non-smokers in 1996, but smoking cigarettes at the time of their second interview

In other words, there is change within the population of smokers, but these cancel each other out to produce an apparently static situation. The likelihood of being a current cigarette smoker at both interviews declined with age, from 34% of men and 38% of women aged 16-24 in 1996 to 16% of men and 19% of women aged 64 and over in 1996. There was no significant difference in the proportion of HEMS respondents in different age-groups who were smoking at one interview, but not at the other. (**Table 2.3**)

2.3.1 Changes in cigarette consumption

Table 2.2 shows grouped daily cigarette consumption; it is possible for a respondent who was smoking only one or two cigarettes more in 1997 than in 1996 to be classified as moving from the 'moderate' (10-19 cigarettes a day) to the 'heavy' (20 or more a day) smoking group. Data on reported cigarette consumption in the two years were combined to see what proportion of respondents were smoking more, about the same or fewer cigarettes at the time of the second interview. Seventy four per cent of smokers had increased or decreased their consumption by fewer than five cigarettes between the two interviews; this is defined as 'broadly the same' for the purposes of the present discussion. About one in six were smoking fewer and just over one in ten smoking more in 1997 than in 1996. There were no sex, age or social class differences in the proportions smoking more, broadly the same or fewer cigarettes, but those who were classified as heavy smokers in 1996 were more likely than others to have reduced their consumption, while smokers who smoked less than 10 a day in 1996 were most likely to have increased the number by the time of the second interview. Thus, for example, among those who were smoking 20 or more cigarettes a day in 1996, 24% of men and 23% of women had decreased their consumption by 5-9 cigarettes a day, compared with no men and 2% of women who had smoked less than 10 a day in 1996. (**Table 2.4**)

2.3.2 Perceptions of smoking behaviour

Current smokers were asked in 1997 whether they thought they were smoking more, about the same, or fewer cigarettes than they were in 1996. Those who smoked 20 or more a day in 1996 were least likely, and those who smoked 10-20 cigarettes daily most likely, to report smoking fewer cigarettes in 1997 than in 1996. Interestingly, when respondents' perceptions were compared with the number of cigarettes they reported smoking in 1996 and in 1997, some of those who were actually smoking fewer cigarettes thought they were smoking more, and vice versa. A half (51%) of those who had increased their consumption by 10 or more a day, said they thought they were smoking the same number or fewer cigarettes than a year ago, while 36% of those who had decreased their consumption by 10 or more a day, said that they were smoking the same number or more. (**Tables 2.5 - 2.6**)

2.4 Giving up smoking

The health benefits of stopping smoking, even for heavy smokers who have smoked for 30 years, are well-documented. Quitting reduces the risk of dying from lung cancer, although there is a time lapse between discontinuing and risk reduction; there is a rapid initial decline in the risk of coronary heart disease in the year after stopping; and the risk of bronchitis and emphysema-related mortality and morbidity is also reduced[7,8,9]. HEMS has therefore included questions asking smokers whether they want to give up and when they intend to do so.

The analysis of the associations between data from the 1996 survey and whether smokers had tried to quit by the second interview was guided by the theoretical models of health behaviour change outlined in Chapter 1. Prochaska and DiClemente's[10] transtheoretical model of change proposes that movement through the stages of health behaviour change is a cyclical rather than a linear process and relapse is the rule rather than the exception. After relapsing, most individuals cycle back into the precontemplation stage; Prochaska and DiClemente found that, on average, smokers made three serious revolutions through the stages of change before they exited into a life relatively free from temptations to smoke. Others get stuck at a particular stage of change. Different processes have been shown to be effective at different stages; awareness raising is most effective at the contemplation stage, while 'self-efficacy'[11], the confidence that one can resist smoking across a range of tempting situations, is important in the action stage of change.

Ajzen's Theory of Planned Behaviour[12], an extension of Fishbein and Ajzen's Theory of Reasoned Action[13], argues that a person's intention to perform a given behaviour is a function of three basic determinants; attitude towards the behaviour, subjective norms and perceived behavioural control. Intentions are seen as good predictors of behaviour. Marsh and Matheson argue that intention has three key components: desire (the wish to give up), resolve (the intention to give up) and confidence.

In common with other surveys[14,15], HEMS has consistently shown that about two thirds of smokers say they would like to give up, and that nearly four out of five have tried to do so at some time[16]. One barrier to giving up is how easy people think it would be to do so. Smokers were therefore asked how easy or difficult they would find it to go without a cigarette for a whole day, which could be seen as a proxy measure of confidence. Although this is

All Change? The Health Education Monitoring Survey one year on

a hypothetical, and therefore subjective question, smokers' perceptions of their own dependence on cigarettes may influence whether or not they try to give up smoking. In all years of HEMS, more than half of smokers said they would find it very difficult or fairly difficult to go without smoking for a day.

2.4.1 Attempts to give up or cut down on smoking in the last 12 months

In line with Ajzen's Theory of Reasoned Action, whether or not someone had tried to give up or to cut down in the last 12 months was associated with intentions expressed in 1996; smokers who said then that they wanted to give up, or that they intended to give up in the next six months were more likely than others to have tried to do so. Thus, for example, 44% of men and 41% of women who said in 1996 that they wanted to give up smoking had made at least one attempt, compared with 25% of men and 19% of women who had not wanted to give up. Similarly, more than two thirds of those who intended to give up 'in the next six months' had tried at least once, compared with less than a quarter of men and 26% of women who said they did not intend to give up 'in the next year'. The proportions who had tried to give up were similar among those who said that they were unlikely to give up and those who said that they did not intend to do so. Marsh and Matheson observed a similar pattern; their questionnaire was more detailed than the smoking section of the HEMS interview, and they were able to see from their data that non-intenders who quit smoking had (at the time of their original interview) more positive attitudes towards giving up than non-intenders who had not quit. **(Table 2.7)**

Smokers in the HEMS sample who said in 1996 that they had tried to give up smoking (at any time, not just in the last year) were more likely to have tried again in the year between the two interviews; 42% of men and 41% of women in this group had done so, compared with only 20% of men and 10% of women who said in 1996 that they had never tried to give up smoking. This suggests that smokers who have tried, but failed on past occasions are not abandoning the attempt, but continuing to try to quit, supporting Prochaska and DiClemente's observation that most individuals do not give up trying to quit when they relapse.

The relationship between the likelihood of trying to give up or cut down and how easy smokers thought it would be to go without a cigarette for a day, was less clear-cut. Men who thought at the first interview that it would be very easy (24%) and women who thought it would be very difficult (27%) to go without a cigarette for a whole day were least likely to have tried to give up in the last year, while men (48%) and women (45%) who thought it would be 'fairly easy' were most likely to have done so. **(Table 2.8)**

Tables 2.7 and 2.8 are based on cross-tabulation techniques, and look at different variables associated with smoking separately. They do not show how much these attributes interact with each other and with other characteristics such as important life events in the last year. It is possible to look at how different factors interrelate by using logistic regression[17], a multivariate statistical technique which can be used to predict the odds of a behaviour (for example, whether a smoker has tried to give up in the last year or not) occurring for people with different combinations of the characteristics under consideration (odds refers to the ratio of the probability that the event will occur to the probability that the event will not occur). The regression looks at the effect of each of the independent variables on the dependent variable, which has just two categories (trying to give up or not) while holding all the others constant.

Ideally, to explain variables associated with giving up smoking, a logistic regression should be used to predict the odds of giving up between the two rounds of the survey. Unfortunately, the number of respondents who had given up smoking in this period and were not smoking at the time of the 1997 interview was too small to carry out detailed analysis, so the dependent variable was taken to be whether current smokers and ex-smokers who had smoked in the last year had tried to give up smoking in the 12 months prior to interview. The independent variables used in the models were characteristics which the literature and cross-tabulations of the HEMS data had shown to be associated with smoking and with attempts to give up; they were:

- age
- whether smokers said in 1996 that they wanted to give up
- when smokers intended to give up
- whether smokers said in 1996 that they had ever tried to give up
- income
- how easy smokers thought it would be to go without a cigarette for a day
- reported levels of stress in the last 12 months

In addition, the following information about events which had occurred in the last 12 months (see Chapter 1) and which might be related to smoking was used:

- whether the respondent reported a serious illness, injury or operation
- whether the respondent or their partner had had a baby or got pregnant
- whether the respondent or their partner had lost their job
- whether the respondent reported serious financial problems and
- whether the respondent reported problems at work

The results are shown in Figure 2.2. The figures in the columns headed 'Multiplying factors' can be thought of as 'weights'; they represent the factor by which the odds of a smoker trying to give up in the last 12 months increase with the attribute shown compared to a reference category[18]. For each characteristic shown, the reference category (shown with a value of 1.00) was taken to be the group of respondents least likely to have tried to give up smoking in the last 12 months.

The variables which were retained by the final model as significant were whether smokers said in 1996 that they had ever tried to give up, whether they wanted to give up, when they intended to give up, how easy they thought it would be to go without a cigarette for a day, reporting a serious illness, injury or operation in the last year, having a baby or being pregnant in the last year (respondent or partner) and reporting financial problems in the last year. The other variables were eliminated from the model. Thus, the odds of trying to give up smoking in the last 12 months for respondents who said in 1996 that they intended to stop smoking in the next six months were increased more than five-fold, while for those who said in 1996 that they had tried to stop at some time they were increased almost four-fold. Having a baby or being pregnant (respondent or partner) more than trebled the odds, while reporting a serious illness, injury or operation in the last year more than doubled them. **(Figure 2.2)**

Figure 2.2 Odds of trying to give up smoking in the last 12 months
Smokers and ex-smokers aged 16-74 who have smoked in the last 12 months

Characteristics	Number of cases	Baseline odds 0.051 Multiplying factors	Confidence intervals
Whether has ever tried to give up smoking (from 1996)			
Yes	709	3.62 *	2.19 - 5.98
No	183	1.00	
Whether would like to give up smoking (from 1996)			
Yes	586	1.32	0.84 - 1.87
No	275	1.00	
Don't know	31	0.42	0.15 - 1.21
When intended to give up smoking (from 1996)			
In the next six months	142	5.46 *	3.36 - 8.84
In the next year	139	2.32 *	1.48 - 3.65
Not in the next year	189	0.91	0.59 - 1.41
Unlikely to give up smoking	422	1.00	
How easy it would be to go without a cigarette for a day (from 1996)			
Very easy	148	1.00	
Fairly easy	222	2.08 *	1.25 - 3.46
Fairly difficult	234	1.50	0.90 - 1.54
Very difficult	288	1.48	0.89 - 2.45
Whether reported a serious illness, injury or operation in the last 12 months			
Yes	86	2.45 *	1.48 - 4.07
No	806	1.00	
Whether had a baby or got pregnant in the last 12 months			
Yes	31	3.54 *	1.51 - 8.30
No	861	1.00	
Whether had serious financial problems in the last 12 months			
Yes	121	1.65 *	1.07 - 2.56
No	771	1.00	
Total	**892**		

* Significant at the 95% level.

The Health Education Authority comments:

Intention to give up smoking within the next six months proved to be one predictor of future behaviour. It is therefore important that health promoters focus on encouraging people to want to change, in addition to simply concentrating on the health effects of smoking.

An interesting finding was the variations in smoking levels over the previous year among those classified as light smokers (that is those who smoke less than ten cigarettes a day), where a small proportion of light smokers in 1996 reported, in 1997, that they had never or only occasionally smoked cigarettes. This suggests a research need to define these smokers in some other way than by the number of cigarettes they smoke and perhaps to see them as 'social smokers'. To define them as occasional smokers has not proved helpful when researching trends in smoking behaviour, or in determining ways to reach this group with health promotion messages.

There was also a mismatch with the levels of cigarette smoking people reported. Some respondents who were smoking more or about the same as they had been a year before, believed that they were smoking fewer cigarettes. If people are unreliable in their own perception of whether they had decreased the number of cigarettes smoked, this must call into question reliance on the importance of advice to cut down as a route towards cessation.

As expected a number of life events also had an effect on smoking behaviour. A few of these, such as a baby in the household, have already proved useful to health promoters. There is an interesting link between other life events, such as having had a serious injury or financial difficulties, and changes in smoking behaviour. This should be further explored.

Notes and references

1. The Royal Society defines objective risk as 'the probability that a particular adverse event occurs during a stated period of time, or results from a particular challenge'. Cited in Adams J. Risk. University College Press (London 1995).

2. British Medical Association. *The BMA guide to living with risk*. Penguin (Harmondsworth 1990).

3. Health Education Authority. *The UK Smoking Epidemic: Deaths in 1995*. HEA (London 1998).

4. Department of Health. *Health of the Nation: a strategy for health in England*. HMSO (London 1992).

5. Thomas M et al. *General Household Survey 1992*. HMSO (London 1993).

6. Marsh A and Matheson J. *Smoking attitudes and behaviour*. HMSO (London 1983).

7. US Department of Health and Human Services. *The health benefits of smoking cessation*. A report of the Surgeon General. USDHHS (Rockville, Maryland 1990).

8. Doll R and Peto R. Mortality in relation to smoking: 20 years' observations on British doctors, in *British Medical Journal*, vol. 2, 1976, pp. 1525-36.

9. Ockene J K et al. The relationship of smoking cessation to coronary heart disease and lung cancer in the multiple risk factor intervention trial (MRFIT), in *American Journal of Public Health*, vol. 80, 1990, pp. 954-8.

10. Prochaska J O and DiClemente C C. Towards a comprehensive model of change. In Miller W R and Heather N (eds). *Treating addictive behaviours*. Plenum Press (New York 1986).

11. Bandura A. Self-efficacy mechanism in human agency, in *American Psychologist*, 1982, Vol 37, pp. 122-147.

12. Ajzen I. The theory of planned behaviour. Organisational Behaviour and Human Decision Processes, 1991, vol. 50, pp. 179-211.

13. Fishbein M and Ajzen I. Belief, attitudes intentions and behaviour: an introduction to theory and research. Addison-Wesley (Boston 1975).

14. Bennett N et al. *Living in Britain: results from the General Household Survey 1994*. HMSO (London 1995).

15. Health and Lifestyles: a survey of the UK population. Health Education Authority (London 1995).

16. In 1995 and 1996, smokers were asked whether they had ever tried to give up smoking; in 1997, they were asked only whether they had tried to give up in the last year.

17. An explanation of logistic regression is given in Appendix D.

18. The odds of engaging in the behaviour in question for people with different characteristics can be calculated by multiplying the baseline odds shown at the top of the table by the appropriate factors. So, for example, someone said in 1996 that they had ever tried to give up smoking and intended to stop in the next six months, and who had had a baby or got pregnant and had financial problems in the last 12 months would have odds calculated as shown below:

0.051 x 3.62 x 5.46 x 3.54 x 1.65 = 5.89

This would give odds of 5.89 that a person with these characteristics would have tried to give up smoking in the last 12 months.

The odds can be converted into a probability using the following formula:

$$p = \frac{\text{odds}}{1 + \text{odds}}$$

so odds of 5.89 can be converted to a probability of 85%, meaning that the model predicts 85% of people with the given combination of characteristics would have tried to give up in the last year.

All Change? The Health Education Monitoring Survey one year on

13

Changes in drinking and drug use

Summary of main findings

- Sixty-four per cent of women and 46% of men reported a weekly alcohol consumption in 1997 which was within three units of their reported weekly consumption in 1996. (Section 3.2.1).

- Respondents aged 16-24 were most likely to report a weekly alcohol consumption in 1997 which differed by more than three units from that reported in 1996; 71% of men and 58% of women in this age-group did so, compared with no more than 55% of men and 41% of women of other ages. (Section 3.2.1).

- Respondents who reported drinking above moderate levels of alcohol in 1996 were more likely than light to moderate drinkers to report a different level of consumption in 1997; more than three quarters did so, compared with less than half of light to moderate drinkers. (Section 3.2.1).

- When asked whether they thought they were drinking more, the same or less than a year ago, 62% of drinkers thought that they had not changed. Those aged 16-24 were more likely than older drinkers to report drinking more than a year ago. (Section 3.4).

- People who thought they were drinking more than a year ago most frequently mentioned 'mixing with people who drink more' (25%) as the reason. Similarly, those who thought they were drinking less were most likely to mention a 'change in work situation or social life' (40%). 'Stress' was the second most frequently mentioned reason for those who were drinking more (18%) and 'cost' for those who were drinking less (15%). (Section 3.4.1).

- Among respondents aged 16-54 who said in 1996 that they had used a drug in the past year, 74% reported using a drug in the last 12 months in 1997. This compared with 4% of those who had not reported using a drug in 1996. (Section 3.6).

- Almost three quarters (74%) of those who reported recent drug use in 1996 said in 1997 that they had used a drug in the last 12 months; 54% were also 'current' drug users, having used a drug in the past month. (Section 3.7)

14

All Change? The Health Education Monitoring Survey one year on

Drinking-Introduction and background

Sustained excessive drinking has the effect of increasing the risk of high blood pressure, strokes and possibly coronary heart disease, as well as being a risk factor for other conditions including cancers and liver cirrhosis[1]. 'Excessive' drinking was defined in the Health of the Nation White Paper as being more than 21 units of alcohol a week for men and 14 units for women. The report set a target for reducing the numbers of men and women who drink above these levels by the year 2005. In 1995, an interdepartmental review of the scientific and medical evidence on the effects of drinking alcohol was published. 'Sensible Drinking'[2] concluded that daily benchmarks[3] were more appropriate than the previously recommended weekly levels since these underlined the need to avoid episodes of intoxication with their attendant health and social risks.

However, in order to maintain comparability with the results from the 1996 survey, the questions used on the HEMS follow-up survey in 1997 reflect the earlier recommendations.

In 1997, HEMS collected data on the estimated consumption of alcohol in units and asked respondents about changes in their drinking in the previous 12 months. This information, combined with that from 1996, provides data for the investigation of changes in alcohol consumption and for the analysis of the relationships between attitudes and intentions expressed in 1996 and any change in drinking behaviour.

3.1.1 Measurement of alcohol consumption

In order to measure alcohol consumption, HEMS uses a similar methodology to that used by the General Household Survey (GHS) and the Health Survey for England. As in 1996, respondents were asked about six types of alcoholic drink, how often they consumed each type, and how much they usually consumed on any one day. From this information, an estimate of the number of units consumed per week can be made[4]. It is known that surveys which collect data on reported drinking behaviour underestimate the amount of alcohol consumed when compared to estimates based on alcohol sales. Respondents may unintentionally underestimate the amount they drink in two main ways. Firstly, they may undercount the amount they drink at home. Secondly, respondents may have problems in recalling the amount they have drunk in any one day or on any one occasion, either due to general memory effects or due to the amount of alcohol that they consumed[5].

The information on estimated units consumed per week can be grouped into an alcohol consumption rating. The terms used for respondents' alcohol consumption levels in this chapter relate to the following number of units per week:

Alcohol consumption level	Number of units consumed per week
Non-drinker	Under one / abstainer
Moderate	1 - 21 units for men and 1 - 14 units for women
High	22 - 50 units for men and 15 - 35 units for women
Very high	51 or more units for men and 36 or more for women

Changes in alcohol consumption between 1996 and 1997

In 1997, the pattern of drinking was broadly similar to that reported by respondents in previous years of HEMS. There was little change between 1996 and 1997 in either the alcohol consumption rating or the mean[6] and median number of units consumed per week. Women's consumption of alcohol was much lower than men's: their mean weekly consumption being 7.3 units, compared with an average of 17.0 for men. About one in four women either drank less than one unit per week or were non-drinkers, compared with about one in eight men. Almost a third of men reported drinking more than 21 units per week compared with about a sixth of women who drank more than 14 units a week. (**Table 3.1**)

A comparison of grouped alcohol consumption in 1996 and 1997 shows that the majority of respondents were placed in the same category in both years. Those who drank moderately in 1996 were most likely to be in the same category at the time of the follow-up survey, with 82% of men and 79% of women also in this group in 1997. Those who were non-drinkers in 1996 were also very likely to report being non-drinkers in 1997, with 73% of men and 78% of women in this group drinking under one unit per week in 1997. Men drinking more than 21 units per week and women drinking more than 14 units per week in 1996 were most likely to be assigned to a different consumption rating in 1997; about half were, compared with a quarter or less of lighter drinkers. (**Table 3.2**)

3.2.1 Changes in estimated units consumed per week

Looking at grouped alcohol consumption does not show by how much individuals have reduced or increased their drinking. Respondents may have changed by only one or two units per week but this could have resulted in their being allocated to a different category. Another way of looking at changes in drinking is to calculate the difference in units between the consumption reported in 1996 and in 1997. These values can then be grouped to provide a meaningful picture of change. The possibilities of problems with recall and accuracy have already been discussed. In order to counteract the possible 'noise' in the data due to these measurement issues and other random variations, a positive or negative difference in consumption of less than four units per week was defined as 'no change'.

Figure 3.1 indicates that the majority of both men and women reported a consumption of within seven units of that which they reported in 1996, although there were a minority whose reported consumption differed widely between the two surveys. One in ten men reported consumption that varied by more than 22 units with roughly half increasing and half decreasing. (**Figure 3.1 and Table 3.3**)

Based on this distribution the differences were grouped as follows:

- at least 8 fewer units consumed in 1997 than in 1996
- 4-7 fewer units consumed in 1997
- 1997 level within 3 units of 1996 level; defined as 'no change'
- 4-7 more units consumed in 1997
- at least 8 more units consumed in 1997

All Change? The Health Education Monitoring Survey one year on

15

Figure 3.1 Changes in alcohol consumption between 1996 and 1997 for men and women aged 16-74 in 1996

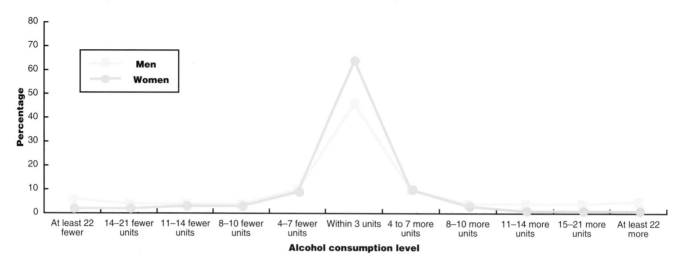

It is generally accepted that there is a seasonal variation in drinking patterns[5] but as the fieldwork took place in May and June in both 1996 and 1997, this variation should be minimised. Respondents' consumption may, however, have changed by varying amounts during the year between the interviews.

Women were considerably more likely than men to be in the 'no change' category (64% compared with 46%). Eighteen per cent of men and 9% of women had reduced their reported weekly consumption by at least 8 units. Women, on average, drank less than men, and, therefore, had less scope to decrease their consumption.

Respondents aged 16-24 were most likely to report a weekly alcohol consumption in 1997 which differed by more than three units from that reported in 1996; 71% of men and 58% of women in this age-group did so, compared with no more than 55% of men in any other age group and no more than 41% of other women. One in four men aged 16-24 (26%) were classified as increasing their consumption by at least 8 units per week but an equal number were classified as decreasing by this amount. Although the percentages were smaller these findings were repeated among young women indicating that this is the age where most change in drinking habits occurs. (**Table 3.4**)

An examination of changes in the number of units consumed by reported alcohol consumption in 1996 confirms the findings shown in Table 3.2. The higher the reported level of alcohol consumption in 1996, the less likely it was that 1997 consumption was within three units of what it was in 1996. Whereas more than four out of five non-drinkers in 1996 and more than a half of moderate drinkers in 1996 reported a 1997 consumption within three units of that recorded in 1996, around a quarter or less of heavier drinkers did so. (**Figure 3.2 and Table 3.5**)

3.3 Intentions and changes in alcohol consumption

In 1996, respondents who drank at least once or twice a week were asked whether they thought they drank:

- about the right amount
- or would like to drink less

Ajzen's model of behavioural change says that attitudes towards a behaviour predict that behaviour[7]. In the case of drinking, the model would assert that a drinker would need to have the desire to reduce their alcohol consumption in order to succeed.

This model appears to have been only partially supported by reported changes to drinking habits between 1996 and 1997. Respondents who said in 1996 that they wished to drink less were more likely than others to report a different weekly consumption in 1997; 77% of men and 72% of women in this group did so compared with 63% of men and 52% of women who thought that they drank about the right amount. But among men, those who wanted to drink less were equally likely to have increased their weekly consumption as to have decreased it (38% in both cases). Among women who wished to drink less a greater proportion had reduced their consumption (46%) but 26% had increased their reported consumption by more than three units per week. (**Table 3.6**)

Figure 3.2 Percentage of respondents whose reported alcohol consumption was within three units of that reported in 1996 by alcohol consumption level in 1996 and sex: adults aged 16–74 in 1996

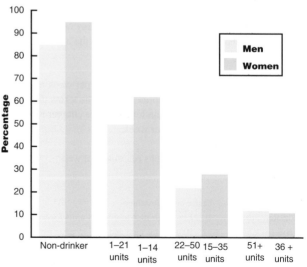

Base numbers are given in Table 3.4

All Change? The Health Education Monitoring Survey one year on

People who said that they would like to drink less were asked which of the following statements best described them:

- I intend to cut down my drinking within the next month
- I intend to cut down my drinking within the next 6 months
- I intend to cut down my drinking within the next year
- I intend to cut down my drinking, but not in the next year
- I'm unlikely to cut down my drinking

The intentions stated in 1996 were compared with the levels of change found in 1997. There were no significant differences between the levels of change for those who said they intended to cut down sometime in the next year (next month, next six months next year) and those who thought they would cut down but not in the next year or those who thought it unlikely that they would cut down their drinking. It is possible that the small numbers involved may have affected these findings. **(Table not shown)**

Perceived changes in drinking between 1996 and 1997

Current drinkers in 1997 were asked about their own assessment of changes in their drinking since the last survey:

'On the whole, would you say that you are drinking....

- more,
- about the same, or
- less than a year ago?'

Just under two thirds of people (62%) thought they had not changed their level of drinking. There was no significant difference between men and women in their assessments, with 13% of men and 12% women who were current drinkers saying they were drinking more and 25% of men and 26% women saying they were drinking less than a year ago. Those aged 16-24 were more likely than other age-groups to report drinking more than a year ago; 33% of men and 24% of women in this age-group thought they were, compared with 3% of men and 5% of women aged 65 -74. The proportions of men and women in the youngest age group who thought they drank less than a year ago were also high. Thus, the self report of current drinkers reflects the findings presented in Table 3.4 that change in alcohol consumption was most prevalent among people in the youngest age-group. **(Table 3.7)**

Respondents who drank very heavily (i.e. 51 or more units for men and 36 units or more for women) in 1996 were least likely to say they drank the same as last year; 38% did so compared with 58% or more of lighter drinkers. Twenty-eight per cent of the heavier drinkers thought they were drinking more and 34% that they were drinking less than at the time of the first interview. **(Table 3.8)**

There was some degree of correspondence between the perceived change and that which was based on change in reported consumption. Men and women whose reported alcohol consumption had decreased by at least eight units were more likely to say that they were drinking less than those whose

alcohol consumption had increased or remained the same as in 1996 (34% for men and 42% for women compared with 24% or less for those in the latter groups). Similarly, those whose reported consumption had increased were more likely to report drinking more. However, comparisons within the change groups showed that while those who were drinking less were far more likely to say they were drinking less than to say they were drinking more, those at the other end of the scale (men in particular) were less likely to be so realistic, with little difference between the proportion who thought they were drinking more and the proportion who thought they were drinking less. For example, among men whose reported alcohol consumption had decreased by at least eight units a third (34%) said they were drinking less and only 8% said they were drinking more, but for men with an increased consumption of at least eight units, 25% said they were drinking more and 23% said they were drinking less. **(Table 3.9)**

3.4.1 Reasons for changes in drinking between 1996 and 1997

Respondents who thought that they were drinking more than a year ago were asked for the main reason they had increased their drinking. The most common reason given was mixing with people who drink more (mentioned by 25% of respondents). Stress was the next most common reason, cited by 22% of women and 15% of men. However, 21% of men and 11% of women thought there was no particular reason for increasing their drinking[8]. **(Table 3.10)**

Respondents who thought that they were drinking less than a year ago were also asked for the main reason for reducing their drinking. The single most common reason given by respondents was a change in work situation or social life, mentioned by 41% of men and 39% of women. Cost was also an important factor (20% of men and 8% of women)[9] and 9% of both men and women mentioned general health reasons. **(Table 3.11)**

Characteristics of respondents whose drinking has changed

The inter-relationships between all the different characteristics which may be associated with changes in alcohol consumption were examined using logistic regression[10], a multivariate technique which can be used to predict the odds of a behaviour occurring for people with different combinations of the characteristics under consideration. Odds refer to the ratio of the probability that the event will occur to the probability that the event will not occur. The regression looks at the effect of each of the independent variables on the dependent variable, which has just two categories (in this case, drinking increased/decreased or did not) while holding the others constant.

Two separate analyses were conducted to investigate the characteristics of respondents whose drinking had changed between 1996 and 1997. The dependent variables used were:

- reported alcohol consumption increased by more than 3 units per week
- reported alcohol consumption decreased by more than 3 units per week

Figure 3.3 Odds of having decreased drinking by more than 3 units a week between 1996 and 1997
People who drank at least once a week, and drank at least one unit of alcohol per week
Adults aged 16-74

Characteristics	Number of cases	Baseline odds 3.07 Multiplying factors	Confidence intervals	
Alcohol consumption in units per week				
1-10 (men) 1-7 (women)	657	0.04 *	-0.46 -	0.5
11-21 (men) 8-14 (women)	606	0.17 *	-0.29 -	0.6
22-35 (men) 15-25 (women)	385	0.31 *	-0.16 -	0.8
36-50 (men) 26-35 (women)	142	0.77	0.23 -	1.3
51 and over (men) 36 and over (women)	115	1.00		
Attitude to own drinking and intentions in 1996				
Wants to cut down and intends to do so:				
Within the next month	65	1.08	0.53 -	1.6
Within the next six months	44	0.48 *	-0.22 -	1.2
Within the next year	40	0.59	-0.12 -	1.3
Not in the next year	23	0.51	-0.38 -	1.4
Unlikely to cut down	155	0.61 *	0.22 -	1.0
Thinks drinks about the right amount	1578	1.00		
Total	**1905**			

* Significant at the 95% level.

The analysis of increase in drinking was based on people who were current drinkers in 1996 while the analysis of decrease was based on those who were drinking at least once a week and at least one unit of alcohol a week in 1996.

The independent variables used in the model were based on the components of the models of behaviour change and those which the literature and analysis of the HEMS data had shown to be associated with change in reported alcohol consumption.

The independent variables used in both regressions were:

- age
- sex
- social class
- economic activity status
- marital status
- qualifications
- tenure
- income
- region
- alcohol consumption in units in 1996
- whether the respondent would like to drink less and, if so, their intentions

whether, during the past year, the respondent:

- reported a serious illness, injury or operation
- or their partner had had a baby or become pregnant
- or their partner had lost their job
- had retired or started a new job
- had married or started a new relationship
- had separated or experienced the break-up of a relationship
- had serious financial problems

The results are shown in Figures 3.3 and 3.4. The figures in the columns headed 'Multiplying factors' can be thought of as 'weights'; they represent the factor by which the odds of respondents increasing their participation are raised with the attribute shown compared to a reference category. For each characteristic shown, one category is taken to be the reference category and is shown with a value of 1.00.

Reported alcohol consumption in 1996 and whether respondents wanted to drink less and, if so, when they intended to do so were significant factors in both models.

No other factors were found to be significant in the model for the decrease of reported alcohol consumption. The larger variation was seen with respect to reported alcohol consumption in 1996 where the odds of people having decreased their reported alcohol consumption were 25 five times less for light drinkers (1-10 units for men and 1-7 units for women) compared with heavy drinkers (51 units and over for men and 36 units and over for women). Intentions appeared to be related to decrease in a 'negative' way; there was no difference between the odds of decreasing reported alcohol consumption between those who said they intended to cut down in the next month and those who thought they drank the right amount. The odds of decreasing reported alcohol consumption for those who said they wanted to cut down but did not intend to do so within the next month were around half to three quarters of those who thought they drank the right amount. This supports the earlier finding that the reasons given for decreasing drinking were mainly circumstantial (change in work situation / social life or cost) rather than due to any self-determined change in behaviour. **(Figure 3.3)**

In addition to reported alcohol consumption in 1996 and intentions, the respondent's sex, age and their household tenure were also significant factors in determining whether reported consumption had increased by more than three units per week between 1996 and 1997. As was the case for decreased alcohol consumption, consumption in 1996 was the most important factor

Figure 3.4 Odds of having increased drinking by more than 3 units a week between 1996 and 1997
Current drinkers aged 16-74 in 1996

Characteristics	Number of cases	Multiplying factors Baseline odds 0.06	Confidence intervals		
Alcohol consumption in units per week					
Less than 1 unit per week	406	1.00			
1-10 (men) 1-7 (women)	1131	2.31 *	1.88	-	2.73
11-21 (men) 8-14 (women)	629	3.10 *	2.61	-	3.58
22-35 (men) 15-25 (women)	394	2.00 *	1.48	-	2.51
36-50 (men) 26-35 (women)	143	1.33	0.70	-	1.96
51 and over (men) 36 and over (women)	116	1.02	0.34	-	1.71
Attitude to own drinking and intentions in 1996					
Wants to cut down and intends to do so:					
Within the next month	65	1.75	1.11	-	2.39
Within the next six months	44	2.80 *	2.10	-	3.50
Within the next year	40	1.96	1.18	-	2.73
Not in the next year	23	1.80	0.77	-	2.84
Unlikely to cut down	155	3.09 *	2.64	-	3.55
Thinks drinks about the right amount	1581	1.51 *	1.22	-	1.80
Drinks less than once a week	911	1.00	0.46	-	1.54
Sex					
Men	1270	1.48 *	1.29	-	1.67
Women	1549	1.00			
Tenure					
Owner-occupier	2104	1.00	0.60	-	1.32
Rents LA	428	1.40	0.95	-	1.77
Rents HA	83	1.90 *	1.31	-	2.50
Rents privately	204	1.00			
Age in 1997					
16-24	155	2.26 *	1.83	-	2.69
25-34	559	1.36	1.04	-	1.67
35-44	695	1.33	1.03	-	1.63
45-54	492	1.16	0.84	-	1.49
55-64	411	1.10	0.75	-	1.44
65-75	507	1.00			
Total	**2819**				

* Significant at the 95% level.

in determining increase. The odds of people having increased their consumption were around three times as high for moderate drinkers (11-21 units for men and 8-14 units for women) compared with the lightest drinkers. For people who wanted to cut down their drinking but thought it unlikely that they would and those who thought they would do so in the next six months, the odds of having increased their consumption were three times those of people who drank less than once a week in 1996. People aged 16-24 had twice the odds as those aged 65-74 to have increased their drinking. **(Figure 3.4)**

Drug use

The White Paper Tackling Drugs Together[11] set out the government's strategy for reducing the health risks related to drug misuse and 'the acceptability and availability of drugs to young people' (this strategy was revised in 1998 in *'Tackling Drugs to build a better Britain'*[12]). Questions on drug use were included in HEMS for the first time in 1996. Respondents aged 16-54 were asked about their use of and attitudes towards non-prescription drugs. The HEMS follow-up allows us to see if drug use has changed in the last year.

In both 1996 and 1997, HEMS included questions designed to measure the prevalence of non-prescription drug use. Respondents aged 16-54[13] were asked to complete this section of the survey themselves on the laptop and were asked whether they had ever used drugs from the following list[14]:

- Amphetamines
- Cannabis
- Cocaine
- Crack
- Ecstasy
- Heroin
- LSD

All Change? The Health Education Monitoring Survey one year on

19

- Magic mushrooms
- Methadone
- Amyl nitrate
- Glues and solvents
- Anabolic steroids
- Tranquillisers
- Anything else thought to be a drug[15]

Drugs were also given their 'street names' to increase the likelihood that respondents would understand the questions. Respondents were asked whether they had ever used any of the listed drugs. Those who had were asked about use in the last 12 months and, if relevant, about use in the last month. As with the British Crime Survey (BCS)[16], this analysis has focused upon use in the last year because it is a measure which is more often reported than use in the last month. Also, because the 1997 survey took place one year on, use in the last year is the most appropriate measure of change between the two surveys.

Drugs were grouped into four main categories, which reflect social attributes rather than pharmacological definitions. These groupings are used to allow comparison to the BCS and between the 1996 and 1997 HEMS[16]. The groupings were:

- Cannabis
- Hallucinants (amphetamines, amyl nitrate, magic mushrooms, LSD, ecstasy)
- Opiates (heroin, methadone, cocaine, crack)
- Other drugs (tranquillisers, glues and solvents, steroids, 'anything else')

3.6.1 Prevalence of drug use

When asked in 1997 which drugs they had used in the past year, 15% of men and 11% of women aged 16-54 had used at least one.

- 14% of men and 10% of women had used cannabis
- 7% of men and 4% of women had used an hallucinant
- 3% of men and less than 1% of women had used opiates

Figure 3.5 Percentage reporting having used a drug in the past year in 1997 by whether used any drug in the past year in 1996 and age

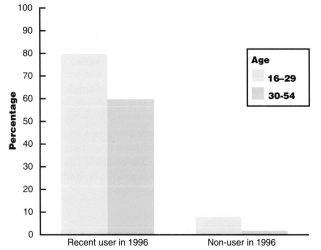

Whether reported having used any drug in the past year in 1996

Base numbers are given in Table 3.15

This pattern of drug use for each category of drug is similar to that found on the BCS, with men more likely than women to report use of all categories, and cannabis being more widely used than other drugs[16].

There were no significant differences in the percentages reporting having used drugs in the past year to those reported in 1996 for either men or women. This compares with the findings from the BCS which showed no change between the 1994 and 1996 surveys for the prevalence of drug use during the last year for the 16-59 age-group[15].

In line with findings from HEMS 1996 and the BCS, the prevalence of drug use was higher among those aged 16-29 than among older respondents. In 1997, thirty-one per cent of men and 24% of women in this age-group had used at least one drug in the last year compared with 7% of men and 4% of women aged 30-54. Among those aged 16-29, 28% of men and 22% of women had used cannabis and 18% of men and 10% of women had used an hallucinant. **(Table 3.12)**

Changes in drug use in the last year

'Recent use' was defined in 1996 as use of a drug within the past year. In general, those who reported recent drug use in 1996 were also likely to do so in 1997.

Almost three quarters (74%) of those who reported recent drug use in 1996 said in 1997 that they had used a drug in the last 12 months; 54% were also 'current' drug users, having used a drug in the past month. There was no significant difference between the sexes, but there was an age difference with older recent users in 1996 less likely to report recent drug use in 1997. Among 1996 recent users, 80% of those aged 16-29 reported having used drugs in the past year in 1997 compared with 60% of the 30-55 age-group. The pattern was the same when respondents were asked if they had used any drug within the previous month: 59% of 16-29 year olds were current users, compared with 40% of the older age-group.

For those who had not reported using a drug in the past year in 1996, 4% had used drugs in the year between the two interviews and 2% had used in the month prior to the 1997 interview. Some of these respondents said in 1996 that they had used a drug at some time in the past. However, respondents aged 16-29 were more likely than older respondents in this group to report recent drug use in 1997, suggesting that some at least began experimenting with drugs in the year between the two surveys. **(Table 3.13 and Figure 3.5)**

Change in drug use was investigated with respect to respondents' attitudes in 1996. In 1996 and 1997 respondents who had used one or more drugs during the past month were asked which one of the following statements best described them:

- I'd like to stop using drugs altogether
- I see no need to stop using drugs at the moment
- I don't see the need to ever stop using drugs

In 1997, as in 1996, the majority of current drug users said that they saw no need to stop using drugs at the moment. A considerably larger proportion of those who saw no reason to stop in 1996 than of those who wanted to stop were still current users in 1997 (75% compared with 49%). However, the latter figure indicates that one half of those who said in 1996 that they wanted to stop were still current users in 1997. **(Table 3.14)**

Comparison of the categories of drugs used by those who were classified as recent users in both 1996 and 1997 with those who had been recent users in 1996 but were no longer so in 1997 (top part of Table 3.15) showed no significant differences for use of cannabis. However, the figures indicated that people who continued to be recent users were more likely than those who were no longer classified as recent users in 1997 to have used hallucinants or opiates in the year before 1996. Similarly, the lower half of Table 3.15 shows that those who were newly defined as recent users in 1997 were less likely to have used these categories of drugs in 1997 than were the continuing users. **(Table 3.15)**

An analysis of continuing users of cannabis indicated that the majority of those who had used cannabis and no other drugs in 1996 were still using only cannabis in 1997. Conversely, a small proportion of those who were using cannabis in combination with other drugs in 1996 reported using cannabis only in 1997. Care should be taken in the interpretation of these results because of the very small sample of drug users provided by this general population survey. **(Table 3.16)**

The Health Education Authority comments:

Ajzens's model of behaviour change (see Chapter 1) was partly supported by the data. Those who reported wanting to change their drinking behaviour in 1996 were more likely to have done so in 1997 than those who thought they were drinking the right amount and expressed no desire to change.

Mixing with people who drink more was the main reason cited for increased drinking by many people. This suggests that health promotion efforts should address the social milieux and acceptability of drinking over the recommended guidelines, in addition to work that concentrates on individual behaviour and benchmarks. The focus on working in health promotion settings in the recent government Green Paper, whilst not specifically citing alcohol, should facilitate this approach.

The sample size of those involved in reporting the taking of any illegal substance, either in 1996 or in 1997, was very small and little change was found in this area of behaviour. However, it is of interest to note that the majority of ever and current users in both years used cannabis.

Notes and references

1. Department of Health. *Health of the Nation: a strategy for health in England.* HMSO (London 1992).

2. Department of Health. *Sensible drinking: The report of an inter-departmental working group.* (1995).

3. The report sets benchmarks for sensible drinking, stating that regular consumption of between three and four units of alcohol a day for men and two and three for women will not accrue significant health risk. However, consistently drinking four or more units a day for men (three or more for women) is not recommended because of the progressive health risk this carries.

4. The method used to calculate the alcohol consumption rating is to multiply the number of units of each type of drink

consumed on a usual occasion by the frequency with which it was drunk, using the factors shown below, and totalling across all drinks.

Multiplying factors for converting drinking frequency and number of units consumed on a usual occasion into number of units consumed per week.

Drinking frequency	Multiplying factor
Almost every day	7.0
or 6 days a week	5.5
or 4 days a week	3.5
Once or twice a week	1.5
Once or twice a month	0.375
Once every couple of months	0.115
Once or twice a year	0.029

The number of units of each type of drink consumed on a 'usual' occasion is multiplied by the factor corresponding to the frequency with which the drink was consumed. In all except the first category, the factors are averages of the range of frequencies shown in the category, for example where a drink was consumed '3-4 days a week', the amount drunk was multiplied by 3.5.

5. Goddard E. Detailed recall of drinking behaviour over seven days. *Survey Methodology Bulletin*, vol. 31, 1992.

6. There were 16 cases which had very large reported amounts for estimated weekly units. Of these cases: three were young women, who drank between 113 and 139 units per week and thirteen were men from all age-groups except the youngest whose drinking varied between 108 and 182 units per week. The pattern of answers these people gave to the drinking questions was consistent and believable so there was no justification for excluding them from the data but the means shown in the report should be treated with caution.

7. Ajzen I. The theory of planned behaviour. *Organisational Behaviour and Human Decision Processes,* vol. 50, 1991, 179-211.

8. The previous section indicates that some of these people were not in fact drinking more which may in part explain the high numbers for whom there was no reason.

9. Although there was a noticeable difference in the proportions of men and women who gave cost as a reason, the difference was not significant because of the small numbers involved.

10. An explanation of logistic regression is given in Appendix D.

11. *Tackling Drugs Together; a strategy for England 1995-1998.* HMSO (London 1995).

12. Tackling Drugs to Build a Better Britain; the Government's ten year strategy for tackling drug misuse. TSO (London 1998).

13. In 1997, these questions were asked of respondents aged 16-55.

14. In 1996, HEMS included the fictitious drug 'semeron' as a check upon false claiming. No-one claimed to have used it in 1996 and so it was not included in the questionnaire in 1997.

15. Non-prescription use was stressed for anabolic steroids; tranquillisers and anything else thought to be a drug by the respondent.

16. Ramsey M and Spiller J. *Drug Misuse Declared in 1996: latest results from the British Crime Survey.* Home Office (London 1997).

Changes in physical activity

Summary of main findings

- In 1997, 26% of men and women were classified as sedentary (i.e. they participated less than once a week in 30 minutes or more of at least moderate intensity activity), while 39% of men and 30% of women were achieving the recommended level of at least moderate activity (five days a week of at least 30 minutes). The figures indicate no overall change in activity levels between 1996 and 1997 among women in the sample but a slight decrease in participation among men. (Section 4.2.1).

- Men and women categorised as sedentary in 1996 were the most likely to have increased their activity; 38% of sedentary men and 44% of women had done so compared with less than one in three men and women who, in 1996, participated once or twice a week in at least moderate intensity activity. (Section 4.3.1).

- Forty two per cent of men and 45% of women had changed their activity group between 1996 and 1997 by more than one day a week. (Section 4.3.1).

- Most change was found among the youngest age-groups. More than half the youngest women had changed groups, with equal numbers increasing and decreasing their frequency of participation. (Section 4.3.1).

- Men and women who had 'left' the sedentary group since 1996 were most likely to have increased their home activities rather than any other activity; 60% of men and 53% of women who were sedentary in 1996 and active at least once a week in 1997 had increased their participation in home activities by at least one day a week. (Section 4.3.2).

- Of those who said, in 1996, that they intended to take more exercise in the next month, only a fifth were more active than they had been at the time of the 1996 survey. (Section 4.4).

- The odds of people increasing their participation in sports and exercise activities were five times as high for people aged 16-24 compared with those aged 65-75. Respondents' intentions (in 1996) to take more exercise and the time period in which they intended to do so were also significant factors in the increase in sports participation. (Section 4.6).

- Significant factors in increasing walking frequency or participation in home activities did not include the intention to take more exercise but did include the frequency of participation in 1996. (Section 4.6).

Introduction

The role of increased physical activity in the prevention and control of chronic diseases is well documented. Physical activity and exercise have been most clearly associated with the control and prevention of coronary heart disease (CHD)[1], hypertension, non insulin-dependent diabetes mellitus, obesity and improved mental health[2,3]. There is also evidence that physical activity may reduce the risk of developing osteoporosis and that muscle strengthening activity reduces the risk of falling and fractures among older people[2]. The role of physical activity in the maintenance of functional ability and the prevention of disability, immobility and isolation also serves to improve the quality of life among older people[4].

The Health of the Nation Physical Activity Task Force consultation paper[5] set out proposals for developing a comprehensive physical activity strategy for England. As part of this strategy the Health Education Authority developed a national promotional programme aimed at encouraging people to be more physically active. The basis for the programme was participation in physical activity at the levels recommended as appropriate for a health benefit:

- five or more occasions a week of at least moderate intensity activity lasting 30 minutes per occasion

  or

- three or more occasions per week of vigorous intensity activity lasting at least 20 minutes per occasion

These recommendations were based on the current US guidelines and agreed by a panel of experts at an HEA international symposium which examined the scientific evidence associated with physical activity and health[6]. This symposium agreed three national objectives:

- to reduce the proportion of the population who are sedentary
- to increase the proportion of the population achieving the recommended level of at least moderate intensity activity
- to increase the proportion of the population achieving the recommended level of vigorous activity[7]

Moderate intensity activity is important because it offers the potential for the greatest health gain in population terms and, at an individual level, represents a more realistic target, particularly for the least active. Population based studies have shown that there appears to be a gradient of benefits as activity increases both in quantity and intensity and although, in general, those at the upper end of the activity scale gain the greatest benefits, in population terms the greatest relative gains are between the sedentary and those who have low activity levels[8].

The levels of physical activity within the adult population (aged 16-74) have been measured by HEMS since its inception in 1995 and by the Health Survey for England from 1991 to 1994[9], but HEMS 1997 represents an opportunity to investigate change in levels of activity at an individual level based on a random sample of the English population interviewed on two occasions one year apart.

This chapter focuses on the analysis of change in levels of physical activity particularly at the individual level, and how it relates to intentions, taking into account theoretical models of health behaviour change which are discussed later in this chapter.

Participation in physical activity

4.2.1   Summaries of activity

- Physical activity as measured by HEMS includes: activity at work
- activity at home (including gardening, DIY and heavy housework)
- walks of 1-2 miles or more
- sports and exercise activities (including cycling)

Two summary measures of physical activity were calculated: one based on occasions of at least moderate intensity activity lasting 30 minutes or more and the other on vigorous intensity activity lasting at least 20 minutes. Moderate intensity activity included brisk or fast walking; heavy housework, heavy gardening or DIY; swimming or cycling (if it did not make the respondent out of breath or sweaty); and some specified occupations. Vigorous intensity activity included running; swimming or cycling (if they made the respondent out of breath or sweaty); and some specified occupations.

The duration criterion of 30 minutes or more used for the summary of at least moderate intensity activity applied only to sports and exercise activities and walking (walks were described as '1-2 miles or more that would usually be continuous walking for at least 30 minutes). Duration was not asked for home activities. Appendix C gives full details of the derivation of these summaries.

The reference period for both these summary measures was the four weeks prior to interview. Data are presented as average weekly frequencies.

As described in Appendix A, not all respondents who took part in the 1996 survey took part again in 1997. There was no significant difference between the 1996 participation estimates based on the responders to the 1997 survey and those based on the non-responders. It is of interest to note, however, that within the group who did not take part in 1997 there was considerable difference between the activity levels of those who asked not to be revisited and those who refused or were not contacted in 1997, with the former group being less active than the latter.
(See Appendix A)

In 1997, 26% of men and women were classified as sedentary (i.e. they participated less than once a week in 30 minutes or more of at least moderate intensity activity), while 39% of men and 30% of women were achieving the recommended level of at least moderate activity (five days a week of at least 30 minutes). The figures indicate no overall change in activity levels between 1996 and 1997 among women in the sample but a slight decrease in overall levels among men both in terms of the proportion who were sedentary (23% in 1996) and of those achieving the recommended level of at least moderate intensity activity (42% in 1996) . The proportion of men and women who were vigorously active at least three times a week for twenty minutes had not changed significantly between the two years (17% and 16% for

All Change? The Health Education Monitoring Survey one year on

23

men and 8% in both years for women). The remainder of this chapter will concentrate on participation in at least moderate intensity activity. **(Table 4.1)**

4.2.2 Participation in different types of activity

Previous analyses of physical activity in HEMS have been confined to investigations relating to overall summaries of activity. Since the 1997 survey is concerned with change, it is appropriate to look in more detail at the types of activity which form part of the overall summary and which are within the individual's power to change. These are sports and exercise activities, walking and home activities. Occupational activity will not be included here. All activities satisfied the criterion of 'at least moderate intensity' **(see Appendix C).**

Comparison of the figures for 1996 with 1997 show that there was very little change in the overall distribution of participation in different types of activity. In both 1996 and 1997, home activities were the most likely to provide both men and women with at least moderate intensity activity; around half the women and just under half the men had participated at least once a week in such activity. More than a third of men and women had participated at least once a week in 30 minutes or more of at least moderate intensity sports and exercise but less than one in five had walked for 1-2 miles or more at a fast or brisk pace with this frequency. There are no published data which are directly comparable with these figures but reanalysis of the Allied Dunbar National Fitness Survey[10] data produced percentages which are broadly in line with the data presented here[11]. **(Table 4.2)**

Change in participation at the individual level

4.3.1 Change in overall activity

In common with other health-related behaviours discussed in this report, the apparent consistency of levels of activity found each year among HEMS respondents masks a considerable measure of change at the individual level. Table 4.3 shows frequency of activity in 1997 by frequency in 1996. Among both men and women most change happened in the frequency groups '1-2 days a week' and '3-4 days a week' (partly by definition since these two groups gave the opportunity to increase or decrease). Men and women in the sedentary group (less than once a week) in 1996 were the most likely to have increased their activity; 38% of sedentary men and 44% of women had done so compared with less than a third of both men and women who participated in at least moderate intensity activity once or twice a week. At the other end of the scale, one in three men (32%) and nearly two in five women (38%) who had been achieving the recommended frequency and intensity of activity in 1996 were no longer doing so in 1997. **(Table 4.3)**

Although occupational activity will not be discussed in detail, it is worth noting here that 7% of respondents were classified into different activity groups in 1997 from 1996 because their occupational classification had changed (either because they had changed jobs or because their self assessment of activity levels at work had changed). Three per cent of people increased into the group classified as achieving the recommended frequency of activity because of their occupational classification and 4% were

classified as no longer achieving this level of activity because of their change in occupational classification.

The analysis of change was intended to look at broad and meaningful levels of change to counteract the possible 'noise' or random variation created by the collection and aggregation of the data. For this reason the measure of change in participation is based on change from one grouped frequency classification to another (as shown in the previous table). This means it is possible for respondents to have changed their weekly frequency but not be classified as 'changers' because they have not changed frequency group. For example, the change from one day a week to two days a week or from three days a week to four days a week does not result in a change in frequency group. However, there is still the possibility that a very small increase or decrease in frequency of participation could result in a change from one broad group to another and this possibility needs to be excluded in the overall definiton of change.

Given the many different questions in the interview used to calculate the number of days of participation, one would not expect the resulting frequency of participation in the four-week period in 1996 and in 1997 to be identical even where respondents' general level of physical activity had remained unchanged. This is borne out by the finding that only 13% of respondents reported exactly the same frequency of participation in at least moderate intensity activity in the four weeks before interview in 1996 and in 1997. Further investigation showed that 38% of respondents had changed their activity participation by less than four days in the past four weeks (i.e. by less than one day a week), so these people were excluded from the group deemed to have changed their behaviour. (Table not shown.)

The summary of change based on these criteria is presented in Table 4.4 which shows that, after taking into account the exclusion of small changes, 42% of men and 45% of women were classified as being in different frequency groups in 1997 from their classification in 1996. Conversely, 58% of men and 55% of women had not changed their overall frequency of activity. Among women the proportions who maintained their frequency of activity increased with age. Over half the women in the youngest age-group had changed, with equal proportions of these young women increasing and decreasing their frequency of participation. Among men there was little variation with age in the proportions who had maintained their frequency of activity. **(Table 4.4)**

Table 4.5 focuses on change at either end of the frequency scale which is of special interest in terms of the objectives agreed by the HON Task Force and the HEA indicators. The figures in bold in Table 4.5 indicate three groups which are of particular importance for health promotion:

- those who were in the sedentary group in 1996 but who had increased their participation and left the group by 1997
- those who had increased their frequency of participation enough to be achieving the recommended frequency by 1997
- those whose frequency of participation was at the recommended level in both years of the survey

There was no difference between men and women in the proportion who had left the sedentary group (both at 8%) and there was very little variation with age given the considerable increase with age in the proportion who were classified as sedentary in both 1996 and 1997.

Younger men and women were more likely than older ones to have increased to the recommended frequency between 1996 and 1997 and were also considerably more likely to have been classified at the recommended frequency in both years of the survey. For example, 43% of men in the youngest age group had maintained the recommended frequency compared with 6% of those aged 65-75, and 15% of the youngest men had achieved the recommended frequency between 1996 and 1997 compared with 8% of men aged 65-75. A greater proportion of men than of women had maintained the recommended frequency of activity which met the intensity and duration criteria (28% compared with 19%). It is possible that this difference was partly a feature of the greater contribution among men made by occupational activity. **(Table 4.5)**

4.3.2   *Change in different types of activity*

Table 4.6 shows the frequency of the three main types of activity in 1997 by their frequency in 1996. It can be seen that the amount of change over this time period varied both with the type of activity and with the frequency of participation in 1997. Among those who were participating less than one day a week in 1996 in any of the types of activity, the majority were still participating less than one day a week in 1997. For example, 88% of men and 83% of women who took part in sports and exercise less than one day a week in 1996 had not increased their participation by 1997. For both men and women, walking at the appropriate intensity and duration was the least likely activity to have shown an increase among people who did not participate in 1996 (92% of men and women who did no such walking at least once a week still did not do so in 1997).

Change was more likely among those who were already participants in 1996. At this disaggregated level of activity summary, decrease in frequency was more apparent than increase and walking was the activity most likely to show a decrease. Among those who were participating in 1996 at the recommended frequency (5 or more days a week) sports and exercise activities showed the highest proportion of 'maintenance' among both men and women (47% of men and 42% of women, who were participating in sports five or more days a week in 1996, reported the same frequency of participation in 1997, compared with 21% of men and 28% of women who had been frequent participants in home activities in 1996). **(Table 4.6)**

It should be noted that the large percentage changes shown among the participants in each activity in Table 4.6 represents a much smaller change in population terms. For example, in overall terms, 13% of men and 9% of women were walking less frequently in 1997 than in 1996, while 8% of men and 10% of women were walking more frequently. (**Table not shown**)

Increases in the different types of activity were investigated with respect to the two overall changes which related to the national objectives, the change from sedentary to a higher frequency of participation in at least moderate intensity activity and an increase in participation which led to achieving the recommended frequency (5 days a week or more). Men and women who had 'left' the sedentary group since 1996 were most likely to have increased their home activities; 60% of men and 53% of women who were sedentary in 1996 and active at least once a week in 1997, had increased their participation in home activities by at least one day a week compared with 24% of these men and 38%

of these women who had increased participation in sports and exercise activities and 20% of men and 16% of women who had increased the number of walks of 1-2 miles or more at a fast or brisk pace. An increase in sports and exercise participation played a more important role for those respondents who had increased their overall participation to the recommended frequency between 1996 and 1997. Forty per cent of these men and 43% of these women had increased their participation in sports and exercise. Home activities also showed a similar increase in participation among these people. **(Table 4.7)**

Intentions and change

The analyses presented so far in this chapter have looked at changes in frequency of participation with no reference to whether these changes were incidental or by intention and no referral to the theoretical models of health behaviour change outlined in Chapter 1. Analyses in the following sections investigate the association between intentions as stated in the 1996 survey, the perception of change recorded in the 1997 survey, external influences and whether people had increased their participation in physical activity.

The analyses will take into account the Theory of Planned Behaviour[12] (which was evolved from the earlier Theory of Reasoned Action[13]) - a behavioural model which states that intentions and behaviour are predicted by two main pathways: the 'attitudinal component' comprising individual beliefs and attitudes and the 'normative' component' concerned with the beliefs of significant others and the extent to which people wish to comply with such beliefs. A third pathway involves the concept of perceived behavioural control which is thought to be particularly important for behaviours which are not under total personal control, of which exercise may well be one. A review[14] of these models in relation to physical activity found that exercise intentions are good predictors of participation and that about 30% of the variance in intentions is explained by the attitudinal and normative components of the models, with nearly all the studies showing that the attitudinal component is dominant.

The Stages of Change Model of Behaviour Change[15] applied to change in exercise behaviour can be used to identify certain stages which take into account intentions and current behaviour[16]. These are broadly outlined as:

- the pre-contemplation stage - those who are not currently exercising and are not intending to exercise in the near future
- contemplators - non-exercisers who intend to start exercising in the near future
- preparation - non-exercisers who are making physical preparations to begin exercising
- action - those who have recently begun to exercise
- maintenance - those who have been exercising for some time

Earlier analysis has identified some of these groups; Table 4.5 looked at respondents who could be said to be in the action or maintenance stages. Tables 4.8 and 4.9 now go on to look at the relationship between intentions and exercise.

Table 4.8 shows how intentions in 1996 related to measured change in participation between the 1996 and 1997. Men who said they would like more exercise in 1996 were more likely to have increased participation than those who did not want more exercise although the difference was not large (20% compared with 16%) and the two groups were equally likely to have decreased their participation. There was no significant difference between these figures for women. Similarly, although there appeared to be a small but significant relationship between stated intentions in 1996 and the proportion increasing participation, in all but the 'within the next six months group' more men had decreased their participation than had increased. **(Table 4.8)**

When intentions were related to changes in frequency of participation in different types of activity, sports and exercise activities were the only type which showed a consistent relationship with intentions. A quarter of men (24%) and women (26%) who said in 1996 they intended to take more exercise in the next month had increased their participation in at least moderate intensity sports and exercise by one day a week or more. This compared with 10% of men and 12% of women who said they were unlikely to take more exercise. **(Table 4.9)**

The results were very similar when this analysis was repeated for vigorous intensity sports and exercise with an increase in participation in such activity among 24% of both men and women who said in 1996 they intended to take more exercise in the next month, compared with 10% of both men and women who said they were unlikely to take more exercise. **(Table not shown)**

It is possible that these findings were affected by the use of the word 'exercise' in the intention question which may be seen as more directly related to sports and exercise participation. Qualitative research conducted during the development of the HEMS questionnaire indicated that when asked to define exercise, people were likely to think that exercise meant 'more than just housework', such as swimming, running and playing sports, although there was the alternative view that exercise came from housework and running up and down stairs all day. Physical activity was thought of as being on the move and included the broad spectrum of activity. However, when asked to distinguish between the two, their explanations were confused and contradictory suggesting there is not a clear-cut distinction between these two terms. **(Full details are given in Appendix B.)**

It should also be noted that the question on intention followed the lengthy section on participation in all forms of physical activity so this should have encouraged respondents to consider the wider spectrum rather than just sports and exercise.

Thus the figures presented in Table 4.9 are likely to represent a real difference in how people change their participation in physical activity, suggesting that activity as part of daily living - walking, gardening etc. is still not used by many as ways of increasing physical activity.

Perceived levels of change in activity

In 1997, respondents were asked whether they thought they had been 'more active', 'about as active' or 'less active than a year ago' to see how their perceptions related to the changes based on reported activity in 1996 and 1997.

Overall, 21% of men and 27% of women thought they had been more active, while 22% of men and 23% of women thought they

had been less active. The proportion who thought they were more active than a year ago was considerably higher among younger men and women than among older people. For example, 42% of both men and women aged 16-24 thought they were more active than they had been a year ago compared with 6% of men and 9% of women aged 65-74. However, the proportion who thought they were less active was also highest among the youngest men and women indicating that these young people were perhaps expressing generally less stable patterns of activity than those in the older age-groups. **(Table 4.10)**

The overall figures for the perception of change among men and women were of the same order as those based on measured change (18% of men and 21% of women had increased their activity frequency while 24% of both men and women had decreased). Comparison of respondents who thought they were more active with those who thought they were less active showed that more of the former group had increased their activity frequency. For example, 33% of women who thought they were more active had increased their activity compared with 14% of those who thought they were less active. But, the figures also showed that within the group who thought they were more active 19% of men and 17% of women had decreased their participation. These differences were seen for each type of activity for women but, among men, were only significant for sports and exercise. **(Table 4.11)**

Contributors to change

When analysing the possible individual contributors to change, it is important to take account of the inter-relationship between all the different factors. These inter-relationships can be examined using logistic regression[17], a multivariate technique which can be used to predict the odds of a behaviour (for example, whether people have increased their frequency of sports and exercise participation) occurring for people with different combinations of the characteristics under consideration. Odds refer to the ratio of the probability that the event will occur to the probability that the event will not occur. The regression looks at the effect of each of the independent variables on the dependent variable, which has just two categories (in this case, increased participation or did not) while holding the others constant.

Three separate analyses were conducted to investigate the increase in each of the three main types of activity: sports and exercise, walking, home activities. The dependent variables used were:

- whether people had increased their frequency of participation in at least moderate intensity sports and exercise (lasting 30 minutes or more) by at least one day a week
- whether people had increased their frequency of walking 1-2 miles or more at a fast or brisk pace by at least one day a week
- whether people had increased their frequency of participation in home activities (heavy housework, gardening or DIY) by at least one day a week

The independent variables used in the model were based on the components of the models of behaviour change and those which the literature and analysis of the HEMS data had shown to be associated with change in physical activity.

The independent variables used in both regressions were:

- age
- sex
- social class
- economic activity status in 1996
- marital status in 1996

in 1996:

- whether the respondent thought they got enough exercise to keep fit
- whether the respondent would like more exercise
- when respondents intended to take more exercise
- whether the respondent was aware of the recommended frequency and duration of activity

whether, during the past year:

- the respondent reported a serious illness, injury or operation
- the respondent or their partner had had a baby or got pregnant
- the respondent or their partner had lost their job
- the respondent had retired or started a new job
- the respondent had married or started a new relationship

whether the respondent saw the following as barriers to exercise:

- not having time
- having an injury or disability that stopped them
- not being the sporty type

In addition, the regression on increase of frequency of sports and exercise participation included:

- frequency of participation in at least moderate intensity sports and exercise lasting 30 minutes or more in 1996
- respondent reported no barriers to exercise

whether, during the past year:

- the respondent had separated or experienced the break-up of a relationship
- the respondent had changed their diet because of weight or health reasons

The regression on increase of frequency of walking also included:

- frequency of participation in walking 1-2 miles or more at a fast or brisk pace in 1996
- respondent reported no barriers to exercise

The regression on increase of frequency of home activities also included:

- frequency of participation in home activities of at least moderate intensity in 1996
- whether, during the past year, the respondent had separated or experienced the break-up of a relationship

The results are shown in Figures 4.1-4.3. The figures in the columns headed 'Multiplying factors' can be thought of as 'weights'; they represent the factor by which the odds of respondents increasing their participation are raised with the attribute shown compared to a reference category. For each characteristic shown, one category is taken to be the reference category and is shown with a value of 1.00. This varied with the type of activity used in the regression.

In the regression on increasing frequency of participation in sports and exercise participation, the variables retained by the final model as significant were: age; when respondents intended to take more exercise; their frequency of participation in 1996; whether respondents saw any barriers to their increased participation and whether they thought they were 'not the sporty type'; and whether they or their partner had lost their job in the past year or had experienced the break-up of a relationship. The largest variation was seen with age, with the odds of people increasing their sports participation being more than five times as high for people aged 16-24 compared with those aged 65-75. For those who said they intended to take more exercise within the next month, the odds of increasing their frequency of activity were around twice those of people who said they were unlikely to take more exercise. (**Figure 4.1**)

The regression on increasing frequency of walking (at the appropriate pace and distance) retained the following variables in the final model as significant: frequency of walking in 1996; economic activity status in 1996; whether the respondent or their partner had had a baby or become pregnant during the past year; and whether in 1996 they thought they got enough exercise to keep fit. Thus, this model did not retain intention to take more exercise, which supports the earlier findings that intention was more likely to be translated into sports or exercise participation rather than other forms of activity. In this model the largest variation was seen with frequency of walking in 1996 where the odds of people increasing their walking were around twice as high for people who walked between one and four times a week in 1996 compared with those who walked less than once a week. For those who (or whose partner) had had a baby or become pregnant in the past year the odds of increasing their frequency of walking were just under twice those of people who had not. (**Figure 4.2**)

The final model for the regression on increasing frequency of participation in home activities retained only three variables as significant: frequency of participation in 1996; social class and age. The largest variation was seen with frequency of participation in 1996 where the odds of people who were participating 3-4 times a week, increasing their participation in home activities were just over half the odds for those who were participating less than once a week. (**Figure 4.3**)

Discussion

An overall comparison of Figures 4.1, 4.2 and 4.3 indicate that the mechanics of change are different for each type of activity with each regression showing different independent variables to be significant. In the case of increase in sports and exercise participation, the variables retained by the regression accord with models of behaviour change - i.e. intentions to take more exercise, current behaviour and perceived barriers to increase. These factors were not so clear for increase in walking and home activities where circumstantial factors seemed to play a more important part. For example, significant factors in the increase of

Figure 4.1 Odds of increasing frequency of participation in sports and exercise activity* by more than once a week between 1996 and 1997; adults aged 16-74 in 1996

Characteristics	Number of cases	Multiplying factors	Confidence intervals
		Baseline odds 0.05	
Age in 1997			
16-24	243	5.18 †	4.69 - 5.67
25-34	648	3.24 †	2.81 - 3.66
35-44	760	3.08 †	2.67 - 3.50
45-54	585	2.43 †	2.00 - 2.87
55-64	479	1.85 †	1.39 - 2.31
65-75	588	1.00	
When intended to take more exercise (1996)			
Within the next month	794	1.97 †	1.72 - 2.23
Within the next six months	658	1.47 †	1.19 - 1.75
Within the next year	312	1.02	0.63 - 1.41
Intends to take more exercise but not in the next year	107	2.03 †	1.52 - 2.54
Unlikely to take more exercise	1432	1.00	
Frequency of sports and exercise (1996)			
Less than one day a week	2182	1.00	
1-2 days a week	611	1.18	0.94 - 1.42
3-4 days a week	249	0.77	0.39 - 1.15
5 or more days a week	261	0.44 †	0.00 - 0.89
Barriers to exercise			
No barriers reported	590	1.00	
Some barriers reported	2713	0.74 †	0.48 - 1.00
'I'm not the sporty type' applies	538	1.00	
Does not apply	2765	1.43 †	1.12 - 1.73
Whether respondent or partner had lost job in past year			
Yes	131	1.60 †	1.18 - 2.02
No	3172	1.00	
Whether respondent had separated or experienced break-up of relationship in past year			
Yes	188	1.49 †	1.13 - 1.85
No	3115	1.00	
Total	**3303**		

* At least moderate intensity for 30 minutes or more.

† Significant at the 95% level.

Figure 4.2 Odds of increasing frequency of walking* by more than once a week between 1996 and 1997: adults aged 16-74 in 1996

Characteristics	Number of cases	Baseline odds 0.04 Multiplying factors	Confidence intervals
Frequency of walking* (1996)			
Less than one day a week	2638	1.00	
1-2 days a week	275	2.25 †	1.91 - 2.60
3-4 days a week	55	1.70	0.93 - 2.47
5 or more days a week	167	0.65	-0.01 - 1.31
Economic activity status (1996)			
Working	2008	1.75 †	1.45 - 2.04
Unemployed	78	1.64	0.82 - 2.46
Economically inactive	1049	1.00	
Whether respondent or partner had a baby during past year			
Yes	105	2.01 †	1.48 - 2.54
No	3030	1.00	
Sex			
Men	1382	1.00	
Women	1753	1.36 †	1.10 - 1.62
Whether got enough exercise to keep fit (1996)			
Yes	1652	1.34 †	1.09 - 1.59
No	1483	1.00	
Total	**3135**		

* At least moderate intensity for 30 minutes or more.
† Significant at the 95% level.

Figure 4.3 Odds of increasing frequency of participation in home activities* by more than once a week between 1996 and 1997: adults aged 16-74 in 1996

Characteristics	Number of cases	Baseline odds 0.21 Multiplying factors	Confidence intervals
Frequency of home activities (1996)			
Less than one day a week	1595	1.00	
1-2 days a week	1214	0.80 †	0.61 - 1.00
3-4 days a week	293	0.61 †	0.26 - 0.97
5 or more days a week	228	0.21 †	-0.36 - 0.79
Social class (1996)			
I & II	1107	1.00	
III (Non- Manual)	778	1.16 †	0.92 - 1.41
III (Manual)	576	1.32 †	1.05 - 1.58
IV & V	692	1.44 †	1.19 - 1.69
Age in 1997			
16-24	246	0.62 †	0.16 - 1.07
25-34	650	1.25	0.96 - 1.54
35-44	770	1.13	0.85 - 1.41
45-54	588	1.07	0.77 - 1.37
55-64	480	0.98	0.66 - 1.30
65-75	596	1.00	
Total	**3330**		

† Significant at the 95% level.
* At least moderate intensity.

All Change?   The Health Education Monitoring Survey one year on

walking included economic activity status in 1996 and whether the respondent or partner had had a baby or become pregnant during the past year; while for home activities, social class and age were the only two significant factors other than current participation. These findings together with those relating to intentions and increase in different types of activity **(Table 4.9)** suggest that models of behaviour change relate more closely to change in sports participation than to activities as part of daily living.

There are, however, some methodological limitations in this data set which need to be noted. First, that the basis of the stages of change model is that changes in intentions precede changes in behaviour. As this data set contains measures from only two points in time it is not possible to investigate whether this is the case. It should also be noted that the interviews took place a year apart while the intentions questions referred to changes within the next month or six months.

The Health Education Authority comments:
It is clear from responses that most respondents still perceive an increase in physical activity as more exercise, rather than as more activities done as part of daily living. However, the increases in physical activity recorded were mainly in daily living activities such as housework and gardening. For a number of health behaviours it has been shown that lifestyle is an important predictor of present and future health status[18]. It is therefore important for health promoters to encourage physical activity as an integrated part of everyday life.

Given the very high levels of variation in participation among individuals it is quite possible that respondents had increased their participation but then dropped back again within the course of the year. If this were the case, then, together with the low levels of 'maintenance' found at the upper end of the participation scale, there is a suggestion that greater emphasis on maintaining increases is needed.

Notes and references

1. Powell K E et al. Physical activity and the incidence of coronary heart disease. *Annual Review of Public Health,* vol. 8, 1987, pp.253-87.

2. U.S. Department of Health and Human Services. *Physical Activity and Health: A Report of the Surgeon General.* US department of Health and Human Services and Centers for Disease Control and Prevention, Atlanta, GA. 1996.

3. Health Education Authority. *Health Update 5: Physical Activity.* (London 1995).

4. Young A. Exercise. In Ebrahim S and Kalache A (eds). *Epidemiology in old age.* BMJ Publishing Group.1996

5. Department of Health. *More people, more active, more often; Physical activity in England - A consultation paper.* Department of Health. 1995.

6. Killoran A et al (eds). *Moving on: international perspectives on promoting physical activity.* Health Education Authority (London 1994).

7. 'Sedentary' people are those who participate less than once a week in 30 minutes or more of at least moderate intensity activity.

8. Blair S and Connelly J. How much physical activity should we do? The case for moderate amounts and intensities of physical activity. In Killoran A et al (eds). *Moving on: international perspectives on promoting physical activity.* Health Education Authority. (London 1994).

9. Colhoun H. et al. *Health Survey for England 1994.* HMSO (London 1996).

10. Allied Dunbar National Fitness Survey. The Sports Council. (London 1992).

11. Health Education Authority. Unpublished data.

12. Ajzen I. The theory of planned behaviour. *Organisational Behaviour and Human Decision Processes*, vol. 50,1991, pp.179-211.

13. Fishbein M and Ajzen I. *Beliefs, attitudes, intentions and behaviour: an introduction to theory and research.* Addion-Wesley (Boston 1975).

14. Godin G. The theories of reasoned action and planned behaviour: overview of findings, emerging research problems and usefulness for exercise promotion. *Journal of Applied Sports Psychology,* vol. 5, pp141-157, cited in Biddle S. What helps and hinders people from becoming more physically active? In Killoran A et al (eds). *Moving on: international perspectives on promoting physical activity.* Health Education Authority (London 1994).

15. Prochaska J O and DiClemente C C. Towards a comprehensive model of change. In Miller WR and Heather N (eds). *Treating addictive behaviours.* Plenum Press (New York 1986).

16. Marcus B H et al. Assessing motivational readiness and decision making for exercise. *Health Psychology*, 11, pp.257-61.

17. An explanation of logistic regression is given in Appendix D.

18. See, for example, Chapters 2 and 3 of this report.

Changes in diet and nutrition

Summary of main findings

- When asked whether they had changed their diet in the last 12 months, 17% of men and 22% of women said that they had made a change to their diet, although these changes were not necessarily towards a healthier diet. (Section 5.2).

- Older people were less likely than younger people to have changed their diet.

- Men in Social Class III (Non-Manual) were more likely than other men to report having a different diet to a year ago.

- The most common changes were eating less fatty or fried food and snacks (mentioned by 8% of men and 10% of women) and eating more fruit and vegetables (7% of men and 9% of women). (Section 5.2).

- Respondents who said in 1996 that they wanted to change their diet in the next month or six months, were most likely to say in 1997 that their diet was different from a year ago. (Section 5.2.1).

- Significant factors in changing diet were found to include: age; marital status; whether the respondent had married or started a relationship; whether the respondent had separated or ended a relationship; and whether the respondent or their partner had lost their job in the last 12 months. (Section 5.2.3).

- The most common reason for making a change was to lose or maintain weight (24%), followed by either a specific health reason, for example, having a special diet due to a specific medical condition (18%) or other health reason (18%). (Section 5.3).

Introduction and background

In the Health of the Nation (HON) strategy, diet and nutrition were identified among the risk factors for the development of one of the main causes of death in the UK, coronary heart disease[1]. Dietary risk factors include: the consumption of fat; obesity; a high sodium intake; and a low consumption of fruit and vegetables. The report proposed targets for reducing the proportion of calories (energy) that the population derives from fat and saturated fat in the diet. Targets were also set to reduce the proportion of the population who are obese.

In order to achieve these targets it was recognised that it would not be sufficient just to cut down on the amount of fat consumed, but there would need to be an overall shift in the composition of the diet. The five main food groups are[2]:

- bread, other cereals and potatoes (starchy carbohydrates)
- fruit and vegetables
- meat, fish and alternative protein sources
- milk and dairy food
- foods containing fat, foods containing sugar

To achieve the Health of the Nation targets, the recommendations were that the main part of a person's diet should be made up of starchy carbohydrates together with fruit and vegetables. Moderate amounts should be eaten from the meat, fish and protein and the milk and dairy food groups. Foods containing fat and sugar could be eaten as part of a healthy diet but should not be eaten too frequently and only in relatively small amounts.

In 1997, HEMS re-interviewed respondents who had taken part in the survey in 1996. The focus of the nutrition section of the 1997 survey was to investigate change in dietary behaviour among those originally interviewed in 1996, and to explore the relationship between these changes and the attitudes and intentions expressed in 1996. It is possible to see the extent to which respondents have made changes to their diet which reflect the recommended nutrition measures outlined above.

Changes in eating habits

In order to see what changes respondents had made to their diet since the original interview in 1996, they were asked the following:

"On the whole, would you say the sorts of things that you eat and drink are the same or different from a year ago".

Respondents whose diet was different were asked for their own assessment of the changes they had made. These may or may not have been an improvement to their diet. Although, as with smoking and alcohol consumption, respondents' self-assessment of their behaviour is not always a reliable guide to actual behaviour change, this question does provide a broad indication of any changes to diet.

The majority said they had not changed their diet in the past year, with only 22% of women and 17% of men saying that what they ate and drank was different from a year ago. Older people were less likely than younger people to have altered their diet, with 10% of men and 13% of women who had been aged 65 or over having

changed, compared with 26% of men and 34% of women aged 16-24. Previous HEMS reports have shown that a high proportion of older people have 'never felt the need to change their diet' or have 'changed as much as they are likely to', so it is not surprising that a smaller proportion of this group had changed their diet since the 1996 interview. These results are also supported by Sheiham et al and the British Social Attitudes Survey of 1989, which found that respondents aged 55 and over had made the fewest changes to their diet in the two or three years before 1989[4]. **(Table 5.1)**

When asked in what ways their diet had altered, most of the changes mentioned by respondents were towards a healthier diet. The two most frequently cited differences were eating less fatty or fried food and snacks, which was mentioned by 10% of women and 8% of men and increasing the intake of fruit and vegetables (9% of women reported eating more fruit and vegetables compared with 7% of men). Women were also more likely than men to have cut down on eating sweets and cakes, with 6% of women compared with 3% of men mentioning this as a change. Five per cent of men and 7% of women mentioned changes which were coded by the interviewer as 'other changes'[3]. Examples of these changes included eating less red meat (1% of men and women); eating a 'sensible' or 'more balanced diet' (1% of men and 2% of women); and eating more fibre or wholemeal bread (1% of men and women). All of the above changes are ones which reflect dietary guidelines. However, some respondents said that the change to their diet had involved increasing their intake of fatty foods, snacks or fast foods, with 2% of men and 3% of women mentioning this. **(Figure 5.1 and Table 5.1)**

Figure 5.1 Reported changes to diet in last year by sex: adults aged 16-74 who had changed their diet

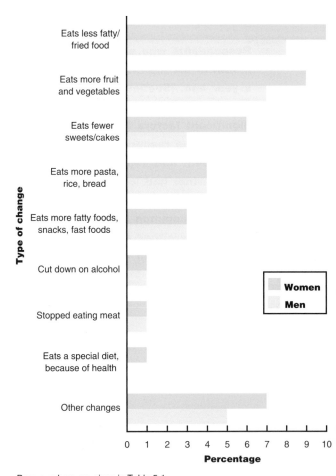

Base numbers are given in Table 5.1

Respondents were able to give more than one answer

Figure 5.2 Odds of an individual changing their diet in the last year
Adults aged 16-74 in 1996

Characteristics	Number of cases	Multiplying factors	95% confidence intervals
Age			
16-24	185	2.54 *	2.06 - 3.02
25-34	615	2.03 *	1.68 - 2.39
35-44	720	1.28	0.93 - 1.63
45-54	555	1.74 *	1.40 - 2.09
55-64	482	1.74 *	1.40 - 2.09
65-75	573	1.00	
Marital status			
Married/cohabiting	1989	1.00	
Widowed/divorced/separated	627	1.57 *	1.33 - 1.81
Single	514	0.83	0.55 - 1.11
Intentions to change diet (from 1996)			
Intends to change in next month	274	2.05 *	1.69 - 2.41
Intends to change in next 6 months	342	2.08 *	1.74 - 2.43
Intends to change in next year	187	1.47	1.05 - 1.89
Want to change but thinks it unlikely	793	1.13	0.84 - 1.42
Does not want to change	864	0.96	0.67 - 1.25
Thinks diet is as healthy as it could be	670	1.00	
Whether married or started a relationship in the last 12 months			
Yes	187	1.71 *	1.36 - 2.05
No	2943	1.00	
Whether separated or experienced the break-up of a relationship in the last 12 months			
Yes	169	1.51 *	1.14 - 1.88
No	2961	1.00	
Whether lost job or partner lost job in the last 12 months			
Yes	122	1.57 *	1.15 - 1.98
No	3008	1.00	
I get confused over what's supposed to be healthy and what isn't (from 1996)			
Strongly agree	97	1.75 *	1.27 - 2.24
Agree	892	1.27 *	1.05 - 1.48
Neither agree nor disagree	359	0.98	0.67 - 1.28
Disagree	1589	1.00	
Strongly disagree	193	1.22	0.84 - 1.60
Number of cases in the model	**3130**		
Baseline odds	**0.093**		

* Significant at the 95% level.

The type of changes made to diets also differed according to the age of respondents. For example, 16% of women and 12% of men aged 16-24 said that they were eating less fatty or fried food and snacks than a year ago compared with 5% of men and 4% of women in the oldest age-group (but the difference was only significant for women). However, 7% of men and women aged 16-24 said that they were now eating more fatty foods, snacks or fast food.

There was no significant difference in the proportion of women in each social class who had changed their diet or in the changes they had made. However, men in Social Class III (Non-Manual) were more likely than men in other social classes to have altered their diet. A quarter of men in this social class had changed their

diet and of those men in Social Class III (Non-Manual) who had made a change, 13% had done so by eating more fruit and vegetables, 10% by eating less fatty or fried food and 10% by eating more starchy foods. (**Table 5.2**)

5.2.1 Attitudes, intentions and changes to diets

In 1996, people were asked whether they thought their diet was 'as healthy as it could be'; or 'quite good but it could improve'; or 'not very healthy'. Those who thought that their diet was unhealthy or could be improved, were asked whether they would like to eat a healthier diet. If they did, they were asked which of the following statements best described them:

- I intend to change my diet within the next month
- I intend to change my diet within the next 6 months
- I intend to change my diet within the next year
- I'm unlikely to change my diet

Comparing the intentions and attitudes expressed in 1996, with whether respondents reported having made a change to their diet by 1997, shows that there is an association between the two. This would fit with Ajzen's model of behavioural change, which says that attitudes towards a behaviour predict that behaviour[5]. If in 1996 people said they would like their diet to be healthier, they were more likely to have made a change by the time of their second interview. Of those who said they wanted a healthier diet, 24% had made a change, compared with only 15% of those who did not want to have a healthier diet. Those who said in 1996 that they did want a healthier diet were more likely than others to report in 1997 eating less fatty or fried foods (12% compared with 5%); eating more fruit and vegetables (11% compared with 5%) and eating fewer sweets (6% compared with 2%).

Respondents who in 1996 intended to change their diet within the next six months were more likely to report a change than other respondents. For example, 32% of those who said that they intended to change next month had made a change compared with only 18% of those who wanted to change in 1996 but thought it unlikely. **(Table 5.3)**

5.2.2 Eating habits in 1996 and changes to diet

In the 1996 HEMS, respondents were asked how frequently they ate different types of food: starchy foods such as potatoes, rice and pasta; confectionery and sweets; chips; biscuits and cakes; and fruit and vegetables, and results from the follow up survey can be used to show whether a change in diet was related to the frequency of consumption of different types of food.

In general, there was little association between the likelihood of making a change and the frequency with which respondents reported eating foods such as sweets, chips and fruit and vegetables. Even among those who had made a change, there was no association between the type of change made and the frequency with which certain foods were eaten in 1996. For example, those who said in 1996 that they ate rice, pasta or potatoes less than once a day were no more likely than others to say in 1997 that they were eating more starchy foods than a year ago, 4% of both groups did so. **(No table shown)**

5.2.3 Characteristics of people most likely to have changed their diet

Tables 5.1 - 5.3 show changes in diet by sex, age and social class separately. They do not show how much these attributes interact with each other and with other variables like attitudes. It is possible to look at how different factors interrelate by using logistic regression, a multivariate statistical technique which can be used to predict the odds of a behaviour (in this case, the likelihood of having altered the diet in the last year) occurring for people with different combinations of the characteristics under consideration. Odds refers to the ratio of the probability that the event will occur to the probability that the event will not occur[6].

Data on attitudes and intentions from 1996 were combined with information on changes from the 1997 survey and a logistic regression model was run to look at the odds of reporting a change to the diet in the last year[7]. The independent variables used in the model were:

- sex
- age
- marital status
- highest qualification level
- economic activity status
- social class
- tenure
- intentions to change diet in 1996

Variables to represent possible barriers to changing diet were:

- total gross household income in 1997
- whether respondents agreed that 'eating healthy food is expensive' in 1996
- whether respondents agreed that 'I get confused about what constitutes a healthy diet' in 1996
- whether respondents agreed that 'the tastiest foods are the ones that are bad for you' in 1996

Variables to represent life events which might influence dietary changes were:

- whether respondents had married or started a new relationship since the 1996 interview
- whether respondents had ended a relationship since the 1996 interview
- whether respondents or their partners had lost their job since the 1996 interview
- whether respondents had experienced financial difficulties since the 1996 interview

The results of the logistic regression are shown in Figure 5.2. The figures in the columns headed 'Multiplying factors' can be thought of as 'weights'; they represent the factor by which the odds of a respondent reporting having altered their diet in the last year increase with the attribute shown compared to a reference category. For each characteristic, the reference category was taken to be the group of respondents least likely to report having changed what they ate or drank in the last year. The reference category has a multiplying factor of 1.00.

The significant variables in the model were: age, marital status; intentions to change diet; some of the life events which had occurred between HEMS 1996 and the follow-up; and whether the respondent agreed that they were confused about what constituted a healthy diet. Once these variables had been included in the model, none of the remaining variables (including sex) were significantly associated with a change in diet. The inclusion of the intention to change diet variable in the model supports the results of the cross-tabulations presented in Section 5.2.1, above; those who intended to change their diet in the next month or six months had odds of changing their diet which were twice as high as those who thought their diet as healthy as it could be. Other results from the regression show:

- If the values of all the other variables were held constant, then the odds of people changing their diet were more than twice as high for those aged 16-24 than those aged 65 or over.

- If a respondent had married or started a relationship in the last 12 months, then the odds of their reporting changing their diet were 71% higher than for other respondents.

All Change? The Health Education Monitoring Survey one year on

- If a respondent had separated or ended a relationship in the last 12 months, then they were more likely to have changed than to have not changed their diet.

The influence of marital status and changes to relationships between the surveys is consistent with a possible change in diet, since a partner is likely to influence what is eaten. Whether a respondent or their partner had lost their job since the 1996 interview was also influential, which can be understood if this had meant a change in household income or in daily eating patterns (e.g. eating at home rather than at work). Being confused over what constituted a healthy diet was one of the possible barriers to healthy eating as identified by Stockley[8]. If a respondent strongly agreed that they got confused over what was healthy then, with other factors held constant, the odds of their changing their diet were 75% higher than for someone who disagreed with the statement.

Reasons for changing diet

Respondents who said that their diet was different from a year ago were asked for the main reason for changing their diet. They gave the following reasons:

- to lose or maintain weight (24% of respondents)
- specific health reason (18%)
- other health reason (18%)
- concerns about food safety (5%)
- cost (2%)
- ethical reasons (1%)

The single most common reason was to lose or maintain weight, which was mentioned by almost a quarter of people who had changed their diet[9]. However, in total, over a third cited health reasons, with equal proportions saying they changed their diet either because of a specific health or an other health reason. Specific health reasons included changing diet because of an allergy or having a special diet because of a condition such as diabetes[10]. Health reasons and weight loss broadly agree with the main explanations given by Stockley for people changing their diet[8]. (Figure 5.3)

There was no significant difference between the reasons given by men and women or between social classes[11]. However, there was a difference between age-groups, with people aged 45-54 being most likely to say that they changed their diet in order to lose or maintain weight (34% of this age-group giving this as a reason). The older respondents were more likely than younger ones to have a specific health reason for altering their diet in the past year, with over a third each of those aged 55-64 and 65-75 giving this as a reason. (Table 5.4)

Figure 5.3 Reasons for changing diet in last year: adults aged 16–74 in 1996, whose diet is different to a year ago

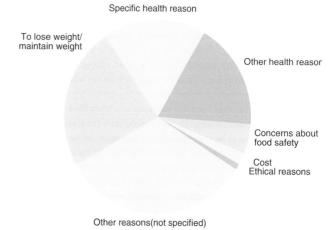

Base numbers are given in Table 5.4

The Health Education Authority comments:

Health messages about diet and nutrition come from a number of different sources, not least the media. With the variation among these messages, which do not necessarily stem from health professionals, it is not surprising that many respondents felt confused about the constituents of a healthy diet. This proved to be a strong barrier to change, and suggests a need to strengthen the visibility and status of authoritative sources of healthy diet information.

The majority of people who had changed their diet had done so for health reasons, for example because of an allergy or health problem or to maintain or lose weight. Health promotion might therefore work more towards stressing the positive effects of a healthy diet for its own sake, if it wishes to encourage healthier eating habits.

All Change? The Health Education Monitoring Survey one year on

35

Notes and References

1.	Department of Health. *The Health of the Nation: a strategy for health in England.* HMSO (London 1992).

2.	Health Education Authority. *Enjoy healthy eating: the balance of good health.* Health Education Authority (London 1995).

3.	Respondents who mentioned an 'other' change that they had made in the last 12 months were asked to say what it was. The answers were coded and seven additional categories created (eats less meat; eats less red meat; eats more fibre or wholemeal; stopped or cut down on dairy food; eats a more sensible or balanced diet; drinks less tea or coffee and more water; and a smaller 'other' category for the remaining codes). However, because of the small number of respondents in most of these additional categories, not all of them are shown separately, but included in 'other changes' in the tables.

4.	Sheiham A. et al. (1987) Food values, health and diet. In Jowell R et al. *British Social Attitudes: The 1987 report.* Gower (Aldershot).

5.	Ajzen I. The theory of planned behaviour. *Organisational Behaviour and Human Decision Processes,* vol. 50, 1991, 179-211.

6.	For an explanation of the methods of logistic regression used on HEMS, see Appendix D.

7.	Because of the small numbers involved, it was not possible to conduct the logistic regression on the type of changes to diets. Instead the variable on whether diets were different from a year ago was used. Not all changes to diets were in the direction of 'healthier' eating.

8.	Stockley L. *The promotion of healthier eating: a basis for action.* Health Education Authority (London 1993).

9.	There was an 'other' code included in this question, for which answers were not specified. Thirty-three per cent of respondents used this category.

10	Interviewers were asked not to prompt respondents at the question on reasons for changing their diet and answers were coded by the interviewer during the interview. Interviewers were asked to use the code for specific health reasons if respondents mentioned changing their diet due to developing an actual medical condition.

11.	Because there is no significant difference between men and women and because the numbers are quite small, data are shown for the sample as a whole and not for men and women separately.

Table 1.1 Characteristics of the sample by sex
*Adults aged 16-74 in 1996**

	Men		Women		All	
	1996	**1997**	**1996**	**1997**	**1996**	**1997**
	%	%	%	%	%	%
Marital status						
Single	26	24	20	18	23	21
Married, cohabiting	67	68	65	65	66	67
Widowed, divorced or separated	7	8	15	16	11	12
Base = 100%	*2044*	*1525*	*2601*	*1923*	*4645*	*3448*
Highest qualification level						
'A' level or above	38	40	28	31	33	35
GCSE Grade A-G or equivalent	38	38	41	41	40	40
No qualifications	24	22	31	28	27	25
Base = 100%	*2037*	*1524*	*2595*	*1922*	*4632*	*3446*
Social class†						
I & II	36	38	25	27	31	33
III (NM)	10	11	34	35	22	23
III (M)	27	28	9	8	18	18
IV & V	18	19	25	25	22	22
Base = 100%	*2043*	*1525*	*2599*	*1923*	*4642*	*3448*
Economic activity status						
Working	70	73	58	60	64	67
Unemployed	6	4	3	3	5	3
Economically inactive	23	23	39	37	31	30
Base = 100%	*2043*	*1525*	*2601*	*1923*	*4644*	*3448*
Tenure status						
Owner occupier	72	75	70	72	71	73
Renting from Local Authority	14	14	16	16	15	15
Renting from Housing Association	3	2	4	3		3
Renting privately	9	9	10	9		9
Base = 100%	*2040*	*1525*	*2597*	*1922*	*4637*	*3447*
Gross annual household income						
Under £5,000	6	5	11	9	8	7
£5,000-£9,999	15	14	18	18	17	16
£10,000-£14,999	16	14	15	14	15	14
£15,000-£19,999	15	16	15	17	15	17
£20,000-£29,999	20	20	18	17	19	19
£30,000 or more	23	26	18	22	21	24
Don't know	4	3	4	2	4	3
Refused	2	1	2	1	2	1
Base = 100%	*2043*	*1525*	*2598*	*1919*	*4641*	*3444*
Standard region						
North	6	6	7	7	6	7
Yorkshire and Humberside	11	11	11	10	11	11
North West	13	12	13	12	13	12
East Midlands	9	9	9	9	9	9
West Midlands	10	10	11	10	10	10
East Anglia	4	4	4	5	4	4
Greater London	13	11	13	13	13	12
Outer Metropolitan and Outer South East	24	24	24	24	24	24
South West	10	12	9	9	10	10
Base = 100%	*2044*	*1525*	*2601*	*1923*	*4645*	*3448*

* 16-75 in 1997.

† Members of the Armed Forces, persons in inadequately described occupations and persons who have never worked are not shown as separate categories but are included in the figures for all persons.

Table 1.2 Life events in the 12 months before interview by age and sex
Adults aged 16-74 in 1996

Age in 1997	16-24	25-34	35-44	45-54	55-64	65-75	Total
Type of event			Percentage mentioning each event				
Men							
Death of close relative or friend	17	27	20	25	25	28	24
Serious illness of relative or friend	11	15	17	17	18	19	16
Family problems	13	13	10	14	14	11	12
Job changes, including retirement	27	25	12	10	9	4	15
Problems at work	12	16	17	21	9	1	14
Serious operation, illness or injury	6	5	7	6	8	11	7
Problems with neighbours	5	6	7	7	8	8	7
Serious financial problems	9	11	6	6	7	3	7
Got married, started new relationship	14	10	6	2	2	0	6
Separation or break-up of a relationship	17	9	4	1	2	1	6
Personal experience of crime	8	6	9	6	2	4	6
Lost job, partner lost job	5	5	3	3	4	0	3
Had a baby	4	11	5	0	-	-	4
Other	6	5	4	2	2	2	4
None of these	25	20	33	34	36	40	31
*Base = 100%**	*123*	*262*	*343*	*295*	*232*	*270*	*1525*
Women							
Death of close relative or friend	20	22	22	22	26	26	23
Serious illness of relative or friend	18	17	20	21	19	20	19
Family problems	26	22	28	30	24	16	25
Job changes, including retirement	34	17	15	11	9	2	14
Problems at work	17	11	15	15	8	1	11
Serious operation, illness or injury	6	9	6	11	9	13	9
Problems with neighbours	9	13	10	4	6	6	8
Serious financial problems	13	10	10	10	4	2	9
Got married, started new relationship	22	11	4	3	1	-	6
Separation or break-up of a relationship	27	11	6	3	2	0	8
Personal experience of crime	13	6	6	5	3	4	6
Lost job, partner lost job	5	8	7	5	3	0	5
Had a baby	4	12	3	-	-	-	4
Other	4	3	4	3	2	3	3
None of these	16	20	25	25	32	35	25
*Base = 100%**	*128*	*398*	*444*	*307*	*278*	*366*	*1921*

* Percentages add to more than 100% because respondents may have given more than one answer.

All Change? The Health Education Monitoring Survey one year on

Table 1.3 Percentage reporting two or more life events in the 12 months before interview by selected characteristics
Adults aged 16-74 in 1996

Sex	Men	Women	Men	Women
			Base = 100%	
Characteristic	Percentage reporting two or more events			
Age in 1997				
16-24	35	52	123	128
25-34	42	42	262	399
35-44	30	42	343	444
45-54	35	41	295	307
55-64	27	27	232	278
65-74	23	21	270	367
Social class*				
I&II	31	38	627	552
III (Non-manual)	37	38	159	671
III (Manual)	34	38	426	162
IV&V	31	39	271	472
Economic activity status				
Working	33	41	1042	1054
Unemployed	39	62	59	43
Economically inactive	31	33	424	826
All	33	38	1525	1923

* Members of the Armed Forces, persons in inadequately described occupations and persons who have never worked are not shown as separate categories but are included in the figures for all persons.

Table 1.4 Life events in the 12 months before interview by economic activity status
Adults aged 16-74 in 1996

Economic activity status	Working	Unemployed	Econonimically inactive	Total
Type of event	Percentage mentioning each event			
Death of close relative or friend	22	15	26	23
Serious illness of relative or friend	16	18	22	18
Family problems	17	30	20	18
Job changes, including retirement	20	3	4	15
Problems at work	18	7	2	13
Serious operation, illness or injury	6	6	12	8
Problems with neighbours	6	9	10	7
Serious financial problems	7	22	8	8
Got married, started new relationship	8	6	3	6
Separation or break-up of a relationship	7	19	4	7
Personal experience of crime	7	4	5	6
Lost job, partner lost job	3	25	4	4
Had a baby	4	4	4	4
Other	4	5	3	3
None of these	28	23	29	28
Base = 100%	2095	102	1249	3446

* Percentages add to more than 100% because respondents may have given more than one answer.

Table 2.1 Cigarette smoking status and consumption in 1996 and 1997 by sex
Adults aged 16-74 in 1996

Year	Men		Women	
	1996	1997	1996	1997
Cigarette smoking status	%	%	%	%
Current cigarette smokers	31	30	29	29
Ex-regular cigarette smokers	28	27	20	19
Never or only occasionally smoked cigarettes	41	42	52	52
Cessation rate*	0.47	0.47	0.41	0.40
Base = 100%	*2042*	*1516*	*2600*	*1919*
Consumption				
Daily cigarette consumption				
- mean	15.3	15.3	2.9	12.8
- standard deviation	8.9	9.6	8.0	7.8
- median	15.0	15.0	11.4	11.4
Weekly cigarette consumption				
- mean	107.3	107.3	90.5	89.7
- standard deviation	62.4	66.9	56.1	54.8
- median	105.0	105.0	80.0	80.0
Base = 100%†	*636*	*439*	*761*	*548*

* Cessation rate = % ex-regular smokers / % ever smoked.
† Smokers only.

Table 2.2 Cigarette smoking status in 1997 by cigarette smoking status in 1996 and sex
Adults aged 16-74 in 1996

Cigarette smoking status in 1996	20 or more a day	10, less than 20 a day	Less than 10 a day	Ex-regular smoker	Never smoked	Total*
Cigarette smoking status in 1997	%	%	%	%	%	%
Men						
Current cigarette smokers:						
20 or more per day	67	21	4	2	-	11
10, less than 20 a day	22	60	20	1	1	11
Less than 10 a day	3	12	54	4	2	8
Ex-regular cigarette smokers	7	6	11	89	-	28
Never or only occasionally smoked cigarettes	-	0	10	4	97	42
*Base = 100%**	*173*	*149*	*115*	*472*	*592*	*1505*
Women						
Current cigarette smokers:						
20 or more per day	67	16	2	1	-	7
10, less than 20 a day	26	66	16	3	0	12
Less than 10 a day	3	13	69	4	1	10
Ex-regular cigarette smokers	4	5	10	90	0	19
Never or only occasionally smoked cigarettes	-	0	3	3	98	52
Base = 100%	*139*	*222*	*181*	*401*	*971*	*1915*

* Includes those for whom number of cigarettes was not known.

All Change? The Health Education Monitoring Survey one year on

Table 2.3 Cigarette smoking status in 1996 and 1997 by age and sex
Adults aged 16-74 in 1996

Age in 1996	16-24	25-34	35-44	45-54	55-64	65-75	Total
Cigarette smoking status in 1996 and 1997	%	%	%	%	%	%	%
Men							
Cigarette smoker in 1996 and 1997	34	30	24	26	26	16	27
Cigarette smoker in 1996, non-smoker in 1997	5	3	3	2	2	4	3
Non-smoker in 1996, cigarette smoker in 1997	5	5	3	1	3	1	3
Ex-regular smoker in 1996 and 1997	4	11	22	35	41	54	25
Never smoked in 1996 and 1997	52	50	48	36	28	24	41
Base = 100%	*141*	*284*	*306*	*292*	*246*	*236*	*1505*
Women							
Cigarette smoker in 1996 and 1997	38	29	27	19	25	19	26
Cigarette smoker in 1996, non-smoker in 1997	3	3	2	2	1	2	2
Non-smoker in 1996, cigarette smoker in 1997	4	4	3	2	0	1	2
Ex-regular smoker in 1996 and 1997	4	10	18	22	26	28	18
Never smoked in 1996 and 1997	51	54	50	54	49	50	52
Base = 100%	*161*	*407*	*432*	*300*	*271*	*344*	*1915*

Table 2.4 Reported changes in daily cigarette consumption between 1996 and 1997 by cigarette smoking status in 1996 and sex
Smokers aged 16-74 in 1996

Cigarette smoking status in 1996	20 or more a day	10, less than 20 a day	Less than 10 a day	Total
Reported changes in daily cigarette consumption between 1996 and 1997	%	%	%	%
Men				
Decreased by 10 or more	7	2	-	3
Decreased by 5-9	24	4	-	11
Changed by fewer than 5 (broadly the same)	62	83	79	74
Increased by 5-9	4	8	14	8
Increased by 10 or more	3	3	7	4
Base = 100%	*160*	*138*	*92*	*390*
Women				
Decreased by 10 or more	15	3	-	5
Decreased by 5-9	23	12	2	11
Changed by fewer than 5 (broadly the same)	59	75	83	74
Increased by 5-9	2	7	11	7
Increased by 10 or more	2	3	5	3
Base = 100%	*134*	*209*	*156*	*499*

Table 2.5 Perceived changes in cigarette consumption in the last year by cigarette smoking status in 1996
Smokers aged 16-74 in 1996

Perceived changes in cigarette consumption in the last year	20 or more a day	10, less than 20 a day	Less than 10 a day	Ex-regular smoker	Total*
	%	%	%	%	%
Smoking more cigarettes than a year ago	13	12	17	18	14
Smoking the same number of cigarettes as a year ago	58	50	46	35	50
Smoking fewer cigarettes than a year ago	28	38	35	33	33
Didn't smoke regularly a year ago	0	0	2	13	2
Base = 100%	*297*	*349*	*248*	*64*	*987*

* Includes those for whom number of cigarettes was not known and current smokers who said in 1996 they had never smoked.

Table 2.6 Perceived changes in cigarette consumption in the last year by reported changes in consumption
Smokers aged 16-74 in 1996

Perceived changes in cigarette consumption in the last year	Decreased by 10 or more	Decreased by 5-9	Changed by fewer than 5 (broadly the same)	Increased by 5-9	Increased by 10 or more	Total
	%	%	%	%	%	%
Smoking more cigarettes than a year ago	6	4	12	31	49	14
Smoking the same number of cigarettes as a year ago	30	38	56	54	25	51
Smoking fewer cigarettes than a year ago	64	58	31	15	26	34
Didn't smoke regularly a year ago	-	-	1	1	-	1
Base = 100%	*36*	*94*	*663*	*62*	*34*	*889*

Table 2.7 Number of attempts to give up smoking and whether has tried to cut down on smoking in the last 12 months by whether wanted to give up and when intended to give up in 1996 and sex
Current smokers and ex-smokers who have smoked cigarettes in the last 12 months aged 16-74 in 1996

Whether wanted to give up and when intended to give up in 1996	Wanted to give up smoking	Did not want to give up smoking	Intended to give up in next six months	Intended to give up in next year	Did not intend to give up in next year	Unlikely to give up up	Total
Whether has tried to give up and number of attempts in the last 12 months	%	%	%	%	%	%	%
Men							
Has not tried to give up	56	75	32	52	80	71	62
Has tried to give up	44	25	68	48	20	29	38
One attempt	25	20	36	35	13	17	23
Two to four attempts	15	4	32	8	6	10	12
Five to nine attempts	2	2	1	4	-	2	2
10 or more attempts	1	-	-	2	1	0	1
Percentage of current smokers who have tried to cut down	57	44	63	68	57	42	54
Percentage of current smokers who have tried to give up or cut down	70	53	78	79	64	53	65
Base = 100%	*274*	*123*	*58*	*69*	*74*	*207*	*408*
Women							
Has not tried to give up	59	81	31	56	74	78	66
Has tried to give up	41	19	69	44	26	22	34
One attempt	24	10	34	28	14	16	20
Two to four attempts	16	8	32	14	10	6	13
Five to nine attempts	2	-	3	1	1	-	1
10 or more attempts	0	1	-	-	1	0	0
Percentage of current smokers who have tried to cut down	62	43	75	72	53	44	55
Percentage of current smokers who have tried to give up or cut down	71	52	86	81	61	52	64
Base = 100%	*339*	*165*	*87*	*76*	*127*	*231*	*518*

Table 2.8 Number of attempts to give up smoking and whether has tried to cut down on smoking in the last 12 months by whether had ever tried to give up and how easy smokers thought it would be to go without a cigarette for a day
Current smokers and ex-smokers who have smoked cigarettes in the last 12 months aged 16-74 in 1996

| Whether had ever tried to give up and perceived dependence on smoking in1996 | Had tried to give up before | Had not tried to give up before | How easy it would be to go without a cigarette for a day | | | | Total |
			Very easy	Fairly easy	Fairly difficult	Very difficult	
Whether has tried to give up and number of attempts in the last 12 months	%	%	%	%	%	%	%
Men							
Has not tried to give up	58	80	76	52	63	64	62
Has tried to give up	42	20	24	48	37	36	38
One attempt	25	14	12	30	23	23	23
Two to four attempts	14	5	9	13	13	12	12
Five to nine attempts	2	2	3	4	1	-	2
10 or more attempts	1	-	-	1	1	0	1
Percentage of current smokers who have tried to cut down	57	39	37	56	62	52	54
Percentage of current smokers who have tried to give up or cut down	70	40	47	73	68	63	64
Base = 100%	*334*	*80*	*74*	*97*	*122*	*117*	*413*
Women							
Has not tried to give up	59	90	65	55	71	73	66
Has tried to give up	41	10	35	45	29	27	34
One attempt	23	7	16	26	17	18	20
Two to four attempts	16	2	17	15	11	9	13
Five to nine attempts	1	-	1	3	-	0	1
10 or more attempts	0	-	2	-	0	-	0
Percentage of current smokers who have tried to cut down	58	44	47	63	56	52	55
Percentage of current smokers who have tried to give up or cut down	68	49	61	73	65	58	64
Base = 100%	*409*	*115*	*84*	*138*	*121*	*181*	*524*

Table 3.1 Alcohol consumption level (AC rating) and mean weekly number of units by year and sex
Adults aged 16-74 in 1996

Year	Men 1996	Men 1997	Women 1996	Women 1997
Alcohol consumption in units per week	%	%	%	%
Non-drinker	7	6	10	9
Under one	7	6	17	16
1-10 (men) 1-7 (women)	31	35	39	41
11-21 (men) 8-14 (women)	24	23	17	17
22-35 (men) 15-25 (women)	17	17	11	12
36-50 (men) 26-35 (women)	7	7	3	2
51 and over (men) 36 and over (women)	7	6	3	3
Mean weekly units	18.0	17.0	7.7	7.3
Standard error of the mean	0.3	0.3	0.2	0.2
Median	12.2	11.4	3.1	3.4
Base = 100%	2007	1517	2560	1921

Table 3.2 Alcohol consumption level in 1997 by alcohol consumption level in 1996 and sex
Adults aged 16-74 in 1996

Alcohol consumption in units per week in 1996	Non-drinker	1-21 (men)/ 1-14 (women)	22-50 (men)/ 15-35 (women)	51+(men)/ 36+ (women)	Total
Alcohol consumption in units per week in 1997	%	%	%	%	%
Men					
Non-drinker	73	3	0	1	12
1-21	23	82	34	11	58
22-50	2	14	56	39	24
51 and over	1	2	9	49	6
Base = 100%	201	822	363	85	1471
Women					
Non-drinker	78	10	1	2	26
1-14	22	79	45	16	58
15-35	0	10	51	25	14
36 and over	-	1	3	58	3
Base = 100%	527	1074	236	48	1885

Table 3.3 Change in alcohol consumption between 1996 and 1997 by sex

Adults aged 16-74 in 1996

	Men	Women	Total
Change in units of alcohol consumed per week	%	%	%
At least 22 fewer units	6	2	4
15-21 fewer units	4	2	3
11-14 fewer units	4	3	3
8-10 fewer units	4	3	4
4-7 fewer units	10	9	10
Within 3 units of 1996 level (=no change)	46	64	55
4 to 7 more units	10	10	10
8 -10 more units	4	3	4
11-14 more units	4	1	3
15-21 more units	4	1	2
At least 22 more units	5	1	3
Base = 100%	*1471*	*1885*	*3356*

Table 3.4 Change in alcohol consumption between 1996 and 1997 by age and sex

Adults aged 16-74 in 1996

Age	16-24	25-34	35-44	45-54	55-64	65-74	Total
Change in units of alcohol consumed per week	%	%	%	%	%	%	%
Men							
At least 8 fewer units	25	17	16	17	14	16	18
4 to 7 fewer units	8	9	12	9	13	14	10
Within 3 units of 1996 level: no change	29	49	45	51	52	46	46
4 to 7 more units	12	10	12	9	8	9	10
At least 8 more units	26	15	16	14	13	15	17
Base = 100%	*137*	*277*	*302*	*291*	*239*	*225*	*1471*
Women							
At least 8 fewer units	16	12	10	7	3	7	9
4 to 7 fewer units	14	11	8	8	7	6	9
Within 3 units of 1996 level: no change	42	59	63	70	77	77	64
4 to 7 more units	11	11	13	10	10	6	10
At least 8 more units	17	8	7	5	2	4	7
Base = 100%	*157*	*400*	*424*	*296*	*270*	*338*	*1885*

All Change? The Health Education Monitoring Survey one year on

Table 3.5 Change in alcohol consumption between 1996 and 1997 by consumption in 1996 and sex
Adults aged 16-74 in 1996

Alcohol consumption in units per week in 1996	Non-drinker	1-21 (men)/ 1-14 (women)	22-50 (men)/ 15-35 (women)	51+(men)/ 36+ (women)	Total
Change in units of alcohol consumed per week	%	%	%	%	%
Men					
At least 8 fewer units	-	8	37	66	18
4 to 7 fewer units	-	13	12	3	10
Within 3 units of 1996 level: no change	85	50	22	12	46
4 to 7 more units	6	11	10	3	10
At least 8 more units	9	18	18	16	17
Base = 100%	*201*	*822*	*363*	*85*	*1471*
Women					
At least 8 fewer units	-	3	40	68	9
4 to 7 fewer units	-	12	16	6	9
Within 3 units of 1996 level: no change	95	62	28	11	64
4 to 7 more units	4	14	8	2	10
At least 8 more units	1	9	8	12	7
Base = 100%	*527*	*1074*	*236*	*48*	*1885*

Table 3.6 Change in alcohol consumption between 1996 and 1997 by respondent's attitude to his/her drinking in 1996 and sex
Adults who drank at least once or twice a week aged 16-74 in 1996

Respondent's attitude to his/her drinking in 1996	About the right amount	Would like to drink less	Total
Change in units of alcohol consumed per week	%	%	%
Men			
At least 8 fewer units	21	32	23
4 to 7 fewer units	15	6	14
Within 3 units of 1996 level: no change	37	23	34
4 to 7 more units	10	12	10
At least 8 more units	17	26	19
Base = 100%	*897*	*189*	*1086*
Women			
At least 8 fewer units	14	32	17
4 to 7 fewer units	16	14	15
Within 3 units of 1996 level: no change	48	28	44
4 to 7 more units	14	11	13
At least 8 more units	10	15	11
Base = 100%	*814*	*166*	*980*

Table 3.7 Perceived changes in drinking in the last year by age and sex
Current drinkers - aged 16-74 in 1996

Age	16-24	25-34	35-44	45-54	55-64	65-74	Total
Perceived changes in drinking in the last year	%	%	%	%	%	%	%
Men							
Drinking less than a year ago	32	27	22	25	21	22	25
Drinking about same as a year ago	34	55	70	67	75	75	61
Drinking more than a year ago	33	18	8	8	3	3	13
Base = 100%	*136*	*270*	*293*	*279*	*225*	*221*	*1424*
Women							
Drinking less than a year ago	37	33	22	22	23	17	26
Drinking about same as a year ago	40	52	65	71	74	78	62
Drinking more than a year ago	24	15	13	7	3	5	12
Base = 100%	*151*	*379*	*407*	*263*	*233*	*290*	*1723*

Table 3.8 Perceived changes in drinking in the last year by alcohol consumption in 1996
Current drinkers - aged 16-74 in 1996

Alcohol consumption in units per week in 1996	Non-drinker	1-21 (men)/ 1-14 (women)	22-50 (men)/ 15-35 (women)	51+(men)/ 36+ (women)	Total
Perceived change in drinking in the last year	%	%	%	%	%
Drinking less than a year ago	24	25	27	34	26
Drinking about same as a year ago	67	64	58	38	62
Drinking more than a year ago	9	11	15	28	12
Base = 100%	*484*	*1880*	*595*	*130*	*3089*

Table 3.9 Perceived change in drinking by change in alcohol consumption between 1996 and 1997 and sex
Current drinkers - aged 16-74 in 1996

Change in units of alcohol consumed per week	At least 8 fewer units	4-7 fewer units	Within 3 units of 1996 level	4-7 more units	At least 8 more units	Total
Perceived change in drinking in the last year	%	%	%	%	%	%
Men						
Drinking less than a year ago	34	25	24	22	23	26
Drinking about same as a year ago	57	63	67	60	52	62
Drinking more than a year ago	8	12	9	18	25	13
Base = 100%	*251*	*155*	*610*	*141*	*232*	*1389*
Women						
Drinking less than a year ago	42	41	24	14	20	26
Drinking about same as a year ago	41	53	69	64	50	62
Drinking more than a year ago	17	7	7	22	30	12
Base = 100%	*148*	*154*	*1074*	*188*	*127*	*1691*

All Change? The Health Education Monitoring Survey one year on

Table 3.10 Main reason for drinking more than a year ago by sex
Adults aged 16-74 in 1996, who said they were drinking more than a year ago

Main reason for drinking more	Men	Women	Total
	%	%	%
Mixing with people who drink more	25	25	25
Stress	15	22	18
No particular reason	21	11	16
Enjoy it	16	12	14
Better off financially	5	9	7
It's good for you/ health reasons	4	4	4
Other reasons	14	18	16
Base = 100%	160	186	346

Table 3.11 Main reason for drinking less than a year ago by sex
Adults aged 16-74 in 1996, who said they were drinking less than a year ago

Main reason for drinking less	Men	Women	Total
	%	%	%
Change in work situation/social life	41	39	40
Cost	20	8	15
Health generally	9	9	9
Specific health reason	4	8	6
Pressure from family	2	-	1
Was affecting my/others life	1	2	1
Pregnant	-	3	1
Advised to by health professional	0	-	0
Other reasons	24	31	27
Base = 100%	154	123	277

Table 3.12 Percentage who had used drugs in the past year by drug category, year and sex
Adults aged 16-54 in 1996

Age	16-29		30-54		All	
Year	1996	1997	1996	1997	1996	1997
Drug category						
	Percentage using any drugs in the past year					
Men						
Any drug	34	31	8	7	15	15
	Percentage using each category of drug					
Cannabis	32	28	8	7	16	14
Hallucinants	18	18	3	2	8	7
Opiates	5	6	1	1	3	3
Other	4	3	1	1	2	1
Base = 100%	417	246	981	729	1398	975
	Percentage using any drugs in the past year					
Women						
Any drug	23	24	4	4	11	11
	Percentage using each category of drug					
Cannabis	20	22	4	4	10	10
Hallucinants	9	10	1	1	4	4
Opiates	4	1	0	0	2	0
Other	1	1	1	0	1	0
Base = 100%	540	326	1205	900	1745	1226

Table 3.13 Drug usage in 1996 by type of usage in 1997 and by age
Adults aged 16-54 in 1996

Drug usage in 1996	Used drugs in past year 1996			Did not use drugs in past year 1996		
Age	16-29	30-54	Total	16-29	30-54	Total
Drug usage in 1997						
			Percentage using any drugs			
Used a drug in the past year	80	60	74	8	2	4
Used a drug in the past month	59	40	54	3	1	2
			Percentage using each category of drug			
Used cannabis in the past year	71	56	66	7	2	3
Used hallucinants in the past year	44	16	35	2	0	1
Used opiates in the past year	14	9	12	-	0	0
Used any other drug in the past year	5	6	5	0	0	0
Base = 100%	*140*	*109*	*249*	*419*	*1493*	*1912*

Table 3.14 Change in drug use between 1996 and 1997 by respondent's attitude to his/her drug use in 1996
Current drug users in 1996 aged 16-54

Respondent's attitude to his/her drug use in 1996	Like to stop altogether	See no need to stop now/ever	Total
Change in drug use	%	%	%
Used a drug in past month in 1996			
and used in past month in 1997	49	75	66
and used in past year, not past month in 1997	23	12	16
and not used in past year in 1997	28	14	18
Base = 100%	*45*	*102*	*147*

All Change? The Health Education Monitoring Survey one year on

Table 3.15 Category of drugs used by change in overall use between 1996 and 1997

Recent drug users in 1996 or 1997 aged 16-54

Change in use of drugs	Used drugs in past year 96 and in 97	Used drugs in past year in 96 but not in 97
Drug category		
	Percentage using each category of drug in past year (1996)	
Cannabis	93	87
Hallucinants	42	26
Opiates	15	3
Other	8	4
Base = 100%	*175*	*73*

Change in use of drugs	Used drugs in past year 96 and in 97	Used drugs in past year in 96 but not in 97
Drug category		
	Percentage using each category of drug in past year (1997)	
Cannabis	90	87
Hallucinants	48	24
Opiates	17	3
Other	7	5
Base = 100%	*175*	*66*

Table 3.16 Change in cannabis use between 1996 and 1997

Recent cannabis users in both 1996 and 1997 aged 16-54

	Past year 1996	
Cannabis use in 1996	**Used only cannabis**	**Used cannabis and other drugs**
Cannabis use in 1997	%	%
Used only cannabis in past year	73	18
Used cannabis and other drugs in past year	27	82
Base = 100%	*95*	*57*

Table 4.1 Frequency of participation in activity by year and sex
Adults aged 16-74 in 1996

Year	Men		Women	
	1996	1997	1996	1997
Frequency of at least moderate intensity activity for 30 minutes or more	%	%	%	%
Less than one day a week (sedentary)	23	26	25	26
1-2 days a week	23	24	30	29
3-4 days a week	12	11	14	14
5 or more days a week	42	39	31	30
Base = 100%	1506	1505	1918	1915
Percentage participating in vigorous activity or 20 minutes or more, at least 3 times a week	17	16	8	8
Base = 100%	1506	1505	1918	1915

Table 4.2 Frequency of participation in different types of at least moderate intensity activity for 30 minutes or more by sex in 1996 and 1997
Adults aged 16-74 in 1996

	Sports and exercise		Walking		Home activities	
	1996	1997	1996	1997	1996	1997
Frequency of activity	%	%	%	%	%	%
Men						
Less than one day a week	62	65	80	83	54	56
At least one day a week	38	35	20	17	46	44
1-4 days a week	26	25	13	12	41	40
5 or more days a week	12	10	7	5	5	4
Base = 100%	1506	1505	1506	1506	1506	1506
Women						
Less than one day a week	65	64	86	86	47	51
At least one day a week	35	36	14	14	53	49
1-4 days a week	29	29	10	10	46	43
5 or more days a week	6	7	5	4	7	6
Base = 100%	1918	1915	1918	1918	1918	1918

Table 4.3 Frequency of at least moderate intensity activity for 30 minutes or more in 1997 by frequency in 1996 and sex
Adults aged 16-74 in 1996

Frequency of activity in 1996	Less than one day a week (sedentary)	1-2 days a week	3-4 days a week	5 or more days a week	Total
Frequency of activity in 1997	%	%	%	%	%
Men					
Less than one day a week (sedentary)	62	30	10	8	26
1-2 days a week	22	39	38	13	24
3-4 days a week	4	14	22	11	11
5 or more days a week	11	18	30	68	39
Base = 100%	*389*	*357*	*180*	*579*	*1506*
Women					
Less than one day a week (sedentary)	56	25	13	10	26
1-2 days a week	26	43	36	15	29
3-4 days a week	6	17	26	14	14
5 or more days a week	12	15	25	62	30
Base = 100%	*496*	*585*	*269*	*565*	*1918*

Table 4.4 Change in activity group between 1996 and 1997 by age and sex
Adults aged 16-74 in 1996

Age in 1996	16-24	25-34	35-44	45-54	55-64	65-74	Total
Change in activity group*	%	%	%	%	%	%	%
Men							
Activity group increased by at least 1 day/week	18	21	17	16	16	20	18
Changed by less than 1 day/week	62	56	56	60	57	55	58
Activity group decreased by at least 1 day/week	20	23	27	23	26	25	24
Base = 100%	*141*	*284*	*306*	*293*	*246*	*235*	*1505*
Women							
Activity group increased by at least 1 day/week	26	22	22	19	21	17	21
Changed by less than 1 day/week	49	52	53	58	60	61	55
Activity group decreased by at least 1 day/week	26	26	25	23	19	22	24
Base = 100%	*161*	*407*	*432*	*300*	*271*	*344*	*1915*

* At least moderate intensity activity for 30 minutes or more. Activity group defined as shown in Table 4.3.

Table 4.5 Changes in frequency of activity by activity group in 1996 by age and sex
Adults aged 16-74 in 1996

Age in 1996	16-24	25-34	35-44	45-54	55-64	65-74	Total
*Change in activity group**	%	%	%	%	%	%	%
Men							
Less than 1 day/week in 1996 &							
Less than 1 day/week in 1997	6	11	12	18	26	28	16
At least 1 day/week in 1997	**4**	**10**	**6**	**8**	**8**	**12**	**8**
At least 1 day/week in 1996	90	79	82	74	66	60	77
Base = 100%	*141*	*284*	*306*	*293*	*246*	*235*	*1505*
Women							
Less than 1 day/week in 1996 &							
Less than 1 day/week in 1997	9	10	10	14	28	35	16
At least 1 day/week in 1997	**11**	**8**	**8**	**8**	**8**	**8**	**8**
At least 1 day/week in 1996	80	81	82	78	64	57	76
Base = 100%	*161*	*407*	*432*	*300*	*271*	*344*	*1915*
Men							
Less than 5 days a week in 1996 &							
Less than 5 days /week in 1997	30	39	47	51	58	78	48
5 or more days/week in 1997	**15**	**14**	**9**	**7**	**7**	**8**	**10**
5 or more days/ week in 1996 &							
Less than 5 days /week in 1997	13	15	15	13	14	7	13
5 or more days/week in 1997	**43**	**32**	**29**	**29**	**21**	**6**	**28**
Base = 100%	*141*	*284*	*306*	*293*	*246*	*235*	*1505*
Women							
Less than 5 days a week in 1996 &							
Less than 5 days /week in 1997	52	48	55	57	69	80	58
5 or more days/week in 1997	**15**	**11**	**14**	**7**	**10**	**6**	**11**
5 or more days/ week in 1996 &							
Less than 5 days /week in 1997	10	17	13	10	8	7	12
5 or more days/week in 1997	**23**	**24**	**19**	**25**	**12**	**7**	**19**
Base = 100%	*161*	*407*	*432*	*300*	*271*	*344*	*1915*

* At least moderate intensity activity for 30 minutes or more. Activity group defined as shown in Table 4.3.

Table 4.6 Frequency of at least moderate intensity activity for 30 minutes or more in 1997 by frequency in 1996, type of activity and sex
Adults aged 16-74 in 1996

	Men			Women		
	Sports & exercise	Walking	Home activities	Sports & exercise	Walking	Home activities
Less than one day a week in 1996						
Frequency of specified activity in 1997	%	%	%	%	%	%
Less than one day a week	88	92	80	83	92	82
1-4 days a week	10	5	18	14	6	16
5 or more days a week	2	2	2	3	2	2
Base = 100%	*1002*	*1223*	*794*	*1288*	*1648*	*883*
1-4 days a week in 1996						
	%	%	%	%	%	%
Less than one day a week	32	49	29	31	49	24
1-4 days a week	56	44	67	61	42	68
5 or more days a week	12	8	4	8	9	8
Base = 100%	*350*	*190*	*630*	*518*	*176*	*887*
5 or more days a week in 1996						
	%	%	%	%	%	%
Less than one day a week	16	45	22	19	53	28
1-4 days a week	37	24	57	38	24	44
5 or more days a week	47	31	21	42	23	28
Base = 100%	*153*	*93*	*82*	*109*	*94*	*148*

Table 4.7 Percentage of men and women who increased their participation in different types of activity by overall changes in physical activity group
Adults aged 16-74 in 1996

	Less than 1 day/week in 1996, at least 1 day/week in 1997		Less than 5 days/week in 1996, at least 5 days/week in 1997	
	Men	Women	Men	Women
	Percentage increasing the frequency of each type of activity* by more than once a week			
Activity type				
Sports and exercise	24	38	40	43
Walking	20	16	27	26
Home activities	60	53	38	45
Base=100%	*123*	*159*	*145*	*198*

* At least moderate intensity for 30 minutes or more.

All Change? The Health Education Monitoring Survey one year on

55

Table 4.8 Change in activity group between 1996 and 1997 by whether, in 1996, respondent would like more and when they intended to take more exercise by sex
Adults aged 16-74 in 1996

Whether, in 1996, would like more exercise and when intended to take more exercise*	Would like more exercise	Wouldn't like more exercise	Intended to take more exercise: in next month	in next six months	more than six months	Unlikely to take more exercise
Change in activity group†	%	%	%	%	%	%
Men						
Activity group increased by at least 1 day/week	20	16	20	22	18	16
Changed by less than 1 day/week	57	59	56	57	58	59
Activity group decreased by at least 1 day/week	24	25	24	21	25	25
Base = 100%	*952*	*508*	*351*	*279*	*172*	*663*
Women						
Activity group increased by at least 1 day/week	22	20	21	26	22	19
Changed by less than 1 day/week	54	56	53	51	58	56
Activity group decreased by at least 1 day/week	24	24	26	23	21	25
Base = 100%	*1273*	*586*	*447*	*384*	*249*	*782*

* 1996 excludes respondents who didn't know if they wanted more exercise.

† At least moderate intensity for 30 minutes or more. Activity group defined as shown in Table 4.3.

All Change? The Health Education Monitoring Survey one year on

Table 4.9 Change in frequency of different types of activity between 1996 and 1997 by whether, in 1996, respondent would like more exercise and when they intended to take more exercise by sex
Adults aged 16-74 in 1996

Whether, in 1996, would like more exercise and when intended to take more exercise*	Would like more exercise	Wouldn't like more exercise	Intended to take more exercise:			Unlikely to take more exercise
			in next month	in next six months	more than six months	
Sports and exercise†	%	%	%	%	%	%
Men						
Frequency increased by at least 1 day/week	16	12	24	15	8	10
Frequency changed by less than 1 day/week	64	64	53	66	68	69
Frequency decreased by at least 1 day/week	20	24	24	19	23	20
Base = 100%	*952*	*508*	*351*	*279*	*172*	*663*
Women						
Frequency increased by at least 1 day/week	21	10	26	20	17	12
Frequency changed by less than 1 day/week	61	71	53	60	68	72
Frequency decreased by at least 1 day/week	18	18	21	20	16	16
Base = 100%	*1273*	*586*	*447*	*384*	*249*	*782*
Walking†						
Men						
Frequency increased by at least 1 day/week	8	10	9	8	9	8
Frequency changed by less than 1 day/week	79	76	75	78	81	79
Frequency decreased by at least 1 day/week	13	14	16	15	10	12
Base = 100%	*953*	*508*	*351*	*279*	*172*	*664*
Women						
Frequency increased by at least 1 day/week	9	11	10	10	10	9
Frequency changed by less than 1 day/week	81	80	77	80	83	83
Frequency decreased by at least 1 day/week	10	9	13	9	7	8
Base = 100%	*1276*	*586*	*448*	*384*	*251*	*782*
Home activities†						
Men						
Frequency increased by at least 1 day/week	17	18	16	17	23	17
Frequency changed by less than 1 day/week	61	59	62	63	53	60
Frequency decreased by at least 1 day/week	22	24	22	21	24	23
Base = 100%	*953*	*508*	*351*	*279*	*172*	*664*
Women						
Frequency increased by at least 1 day/week	17	18	14	20	19	17
Frequency changed by less than 1 day/week	60	57	61	58	60	58
Frequency decreased by at least 1 day/week	23	25	25	22	21	25
Base = 100%	*1276*	*586*	*448*	*384*	*251*	*782*

* 1996 excludes respondents who didn't know if they wanted more exercise.

† At least moderate intensity for 30 minutes or more.

All Change? The Health Education Monitoring Survey one year on

57

Table 4.10 Perceived change in activity comparing 1997 with a year ago by age and sex
Adults aged 16-74 in 1996

Age in 1996	16-24	25-34	35-44	45-54	55-64	65-74	Total
Perceived change in activity	%	%	%	%	%	%	%
Men							
More active than a year ago	42	27	20	14	11	6	21
About as active as a year ago	30	51	62	64	69	71	57
Less active than a year ago	28	22	17	22	20	23	22
Base = 100%	*140*	*283*	*300*	*285*	*236*	*222*	*1466*
Women							
More active than a year ago	42	40	26	19	19	9	27
About as active as a year ago	30	38	49	61	64	69	50
Less active than a year ago	28	22	26	20	17	22	23
Base = 100%	*161*	*402*	*427*	*298*	*259*	*317*	*1864*

Table 4.11 Perceived change in activity comparing 1997 with a year ago by change in reported activity* and sex
Adults aged 16-74 in 1996

Perceived change in activity	Men			Women		
	More active than a year ago	About the same as a year ago	Less active than a year ago	More active than a year ago	About the same as a year ago	Less active than a year ago
	%	%	%	%	%	%
Change in activity group*						
Activity group increased by at least 1 day/week	24	18	14	33	19	14
Changed by less than 1 day/week	56	59	55	50	59	52
Activity group decreased by at least 1 day/week	19	23	30	17	22	35
Base = 100%	*276*	*868*	*321*	*465*	*965*	*434*
Change in frequency of sports and exercise†						
Frequency increased by at least 1 day/week	27	11	12	33	13	11
Frequency changed by less than 1 day/week	48	73	59	52	71	61
Frequency decreased by at least 1 day/week	25	16	30	15	16	28
Base = 100%	*276*	*868*	*321*	*465*	*965*	*434*
Change in frequency of walking†						
Frequency increased by at least 1 day/week	10	8	7	15	9	5
Frequency changed by less than 1 day/week	73	80	80	74	82	87
Frequency decreased by at least 1 day/week	17	12	13	11	9	8
Base = 100%	*276*	*869*	*321*	*465*	*965*	*434*
Change in frequency of home activities†						
Frequency increased by at least 1 day/week	17	19	14	21	17	14
Frequency changed by less than 1 day/week	58	58	68	58	59	60
Frequency decreased by at least 1 day/week	25	23	18	21	24	25
Base = 100%	*276*	*869*	*321*	*465*	*965*	*434*

* Activity group defined as shown in Table 4.4

† At least moderate intensity for 30 minutes or more.

All Change? The Health Education Monitoring Survey one year on

Table 5.1 Changes to diet in the last year by age and sex
Adults aged 16-74 in 1996

Age in 1996	16-24	25-34	35-44	45-54	55-64	65-74	Total
How diet has changed in last year			Percentage making each change				
Men							
Has not changed diet	74	79	86	84	84	90	83
Eats less fatty/fried foods	12	10	7	7	8	5	8
Eats more fruit and vegetables	9	9	4	6	8	2	7
Eats more pasta, rice, bread	7	4	2	5	4	1	4
Eats fewer sweets/cakes	6	3	2	1	5	2	3
Eats more fatty foods, snacks, fast foods	7	2	3	0	1	1	2
Stopped eating meat	1	0	0	1	1	0	1
Cut down on alcohol	1	1	1	1	1	-	1
Eats a special diet, because of health	-	-	-	0	0	1	0
Other changes	4	7	5	6	3	4	5
Including:							
Eats less red meat	1	1	0	2	-	1	1
Eats a more sensible, balanced diet	1	1	2	0	0	0	1
Eats more fibre, wholemeal food	-	2	0	1	-	1	1
*Base**	*141*	*290*	*310*	*296*	*247*	*235*	*1519*
Women							
Has not changed diet	66	76	82	80	80	87	78
Eats less fatty/fried foods	16	10	9	10	10	4	10
Eats more fruit and vegetables	18	10	7	11	7	4	9
Eats more pasta, rice, bread	8	5	3	3	3	1	4
Eats fewer sweets/cakes	10	6	5	6	4	2	6
Eats more fatty foods, snacks, fast foods	7	4	2	1	2	1	3
Stopped eating meat	2	1	1	1	2	0	1
Cut down on alcohol	4	2	1	0	0	0	1
Eats a special diet, because of health	0	-	1	1	1	1	1
Other changes	12	6	6	7	8	4	7
Including:							
Eats less red meat	2	-	1	1	2	0	1
Eats a more sensible, balanced diet	4	2	1	1	-	1	2
Eats more fibre, wholemeal food	-	0	0	2	1	-	1
*Base**	*162*	*406*	*433*	*301*	*273*	*342*	*1917*

* Percentages total more than 100% as respondents could give more than one answer.

Table 5.2 Changes to diet in the last year by social class based on own current or last job, and sex
Adults aged 16-74 in 1996

Social class	I & II	III(NM)	III(M)	IV & V	Total*
How diet has changed in last year	Percentage making each change				
Men					
Has not changed diet	87	75	82	83	83
Eats less fatty/fried foods	6	10	10	7	8
Eats more fruit and vegetables	5	13	6	7	7
Eats more pasta, rice, bread	1	10	4	4	4
Eats fewer sweets/cakes	3	5	4	2	3
Eats more fatty foods, snacks, fast foods	2	3	2	2	3
Stopped eating meat	0	0	0	2	1
Cut down on alcohol	1	2	1	0	1
Eats a special diet, because of health	0	-	0	0	0
Other changes	5	6	5	4	5
Including:					
Eats less red meat	0	1	1	1	1
Eats a more sensible, balanced diet	1	1	1	0	1
Eats more fibre, wholemeal food	-	2	0	1	1
Base †	*625*	*159*	*426*	*268*	*1519*
Women					
Has not changed diet	78	78	77	79	78
Eats less fatty/fried foods	10	11	10	10	10
Eats more fruit and vegetables	11	9	10	9	9
Eats more pasta, rice, bread	5	4	5	4	4
Eats fewer sweets/cakes	6	6	7	5	6
Eats more fatty foods, snacks, fast foods	3	2	3	3	3
Stopped eating meat	1	1	2	1	1
Cut down on alcohol	2	2	1	1	1
Eats a special diet, because of health	1	0	-	1	1
Other changes	7	7	7	7	7
Including:					
Eats less red meat	2	1	1	1	1
Eats a more sensible, balanced diet	2	1	1	1	2
Eats more fibre, wholemeal food	0	1	1	0	1
Base †	*552*	*669*	*161*	*472*	*1917*

* Members of the Armed Forces, persons in inadequately described occupations and persons who have never worked are not shown as separate categories but are included in the figures for all persons.

† Percentages total more than 100% as respondents could give more than one answer.

Table 5.3 Changes to diet by 1996 intentions to change diet
Adults aged 16-74, who in 1996 said their diet was not as healthy as it could be

In 1996, intentions to change diet	Whether wanted diet to be healthier		When intended to change				Total*
	Yes	No	Next month	Next 6 months	Next year	Wants to change but unlikely	
How diet has changed in last year			Percentage making each change				
Has not changed diet	76	85	68	70	75	82	79
Eats less fatty/fried food	12	5	14	18	16	8	10
Eats more fruit and vegetables	11	5	14	17	9	7	8
Eats more pasta, rice, bread	5	3	7	8	3	3	4
Eats fewer sweets/cakes	6	2	10	9	7	3	5
Eats more fatty foods, snacks, fast foods	3	5	14	18	16	8	3
Stopped eating meat	1	0	3	0	0	1	1
Cut down on alcohol	2	1	3	2	2	1	1
Eats a special diet, because of health	0	0	0	0	0	0	0
Other changes	8	4	10	11	9	6	7
Base †	1703	914	293	369	197	837	2687

* Total includes a small number of respondents who did not know if they wanted to have a healthier diet.

† Percentages total more than 100% as respondents could give more than one answer.

Table 5.4 Reasons for changing diet in the last year by age
Adults aged 16-74 in 1996

Age in 1996	16-24	25-34	35-44	45-54	55-64	65-74	Total
Why changed diet in last year	%	%	%	%	%	%	%
To lose weight/maintain weight	19	27	22	34	20	17	24
Specific health reason	6	12	19	18	38	34	18
Other health reason	22	16	15	22	15	14	18
Concerns about food safety	5	4	4	5	4	8	5
Cost	3	3	1	-	1	2	2
Ethical reasons	1	2	1	-	1	-	1
Other reasons (not specified)	44	36	38	20	20	24	33
Base = 100%	89	160	124	118	97	64	652

Part B - *Sexual behaviour and sun exposure tables*

Tables on sexual health and sun exposure

The 1997 survey included questions on sexual health and sun exposure. The results are not reported in the main body of the report but for completeness tables are included showing the situation in 1997

Table 6.1 Age at first intercourse by age and sex
Adults aged 16-54 in 1997

Age in 1997	16-19	20-24	25-34	35-44	45-55	Total
Age at first intercourse	%	%	%	%	%	%
Men						
Never had a sexual partner	31	10	4	1	1	6
Under 16	25	20	26	21	13	20
16-17	39	48	33	36	27	34
18-19	6	16	21	23	29	22
20-24	-	5	12	16	23	14
25 or over	-	-	3	3	7	4
Base = 100%	*55*	*59*	*250*	*319*	*298*	*981*
Mean (average) age	15.8	16.3	17.2	17.5	18.9	17.6
Standard error of the mean	0.12	0.14	0.12	0.12	0.17	0.07
5th percentile	13	13	13	13	14	14
10th percentile	14	14	14	15	15	14
Median age	16	16	17	17	18	17
90th percentile	17	19	21	21	24	21
95th percentile	19	20	23	22	26	23
Base = 100%*	*40*	*54*	*236*	*313*	*292*	*935*
Women						
Never had a sexual partner	24	8	2	2	1	4
Under 16	38	25	17	10	3	14
16-17	24	30	41	40	27	35
18-19	13	24	26	29	31	27
20-24	-	13	13	15	31	17
25 or over	-	-	1	4	7	3
Base = 100%	*33*	*83*	*373*	*411*	*308*	*1208*
Mean (average) age	15.3	17	17.2	17.9	19.4	17.9
Standard error of the mean	0.21	0.14	0.09	0.11	0.17	0.07
5th percentile	12	14	14	15	16	14
10th percentile	13	15	15	15	16	15
Median age	15	17	17	17	19	17
90th percentile	18	20	20	21	23	21
95th percentile	18	21	21	24	25	23
Base = 100%*	*25*	*79*	*367*	*403*	*301*	*1175*

* Excludes those reporting no sexual partner.

All Change? The Health Education Monitoring Survey one year on

Table 6.2 Number of sexual partners in the last 12 months by year and sex
Adults aged 16-54 in 1996

	Men		Women	
			1996-1997 *	
Year	1996	1997	1996	1997
Number of sexual partners in the last 12 months	%	%	%	%
None	14	13	12	13
One	69	71	78	78
Two	7	6	5	5
Three to four	5	6	3	3
Five to nine	2	3	1	2
Ten or more	1	1	0	0
Base = 100%	*1375*	*982*	*1716*	*1215*
Median	1	1	1	1
95th percentile	4	4	2	3
Base = 100%†	*1173*	*848*	*1484*	*1046*

* Proportions differ from those shown in the 1995 report because they exclude married, cohabiting, widowed, divorced and separated respondents who said they had never had a sexual partner.

† Excludes respondents who did not report a sexual partner in the last year.

Table 6.3 Number of sexual partners in the last 12 months in 1997 by number of sexual partners in the last 12 months in 1996 and sex
Adults aged 16-54 in 1996

Number of sexual partners in the last 12 months in 1996	No sexual partner in the last 12 months	One	Two or more	Total
Number of sexual partners in the last 12 months in 1997	%	%	%	%
Men				
No sexual partner in the last 12 months	61	4	5	13
One	27	89	33	71
Two	12	7	62	16
Base = 100%	*139*	*663*	*143*	*945*
Women				
No sexual partner in the last 12 months	71	4	6	13
One	22	91	38	78
Two	8	5	56	10
Base = 100%	*157*	*921*	*111*	*1189*

Table 6.4 Number of sexual partners in the last 12 months in 1997 by assessment of risk of getting HIV (the AIDS virus) in 1996 and sex
Adults aged 16-54 in 1996

Assessment of risk of getting HIV (the AIDS virus) in 1996	Very or quite high	Low	No risk	Total
Number of sexual partners in the last 12 months in 1997	%	%	%	%
Men				
No sexual partner in the last 12 months	18	14	8	13
One	44	69	85	71
Two	38	17	7	16
Base = 100%	*86*	*529*	*290*	*954*
Women				
No sexual partner in the last 12 months	8	11	17	13
One	66	76	80	78
Two	26	12	3	10
Base = 100%	*78*	*698*	*366*	*1199*

Table 6.5 Number of sexual partners in the last 12 months in 1997 by assessment of risk of getting another sexually transmitted disease in 1996 and sex
Adults aged 16-54 in 1996

Assessment of risk of getting another sexually transmitted disease in 1996	Very or quite high	Low	No risk	Total
Number of sexual partners in the last 12 months in 1997	%	%	%	%
Men				
No sexual partner in the last 12 months	18	14	9	13
One	38	69	83	71
Two	44	17	8	16
Base = 100%	*74*	*510*	*332*	*954*
Women				
No sexual partner in the last 12 months	8	10	17	13
One	55	80	80	78
Two	37	11	3	10
Base = 100%	*70*	*698*	*394*	*1199*

Table 6.6 Respondents' assessment of the likelihood of 'someone like me getting HIV (the AIDS virus)' by year and sex
Adults aged 16-54 in 1996

	Men		Women	
	1996-1997			
Year	1996	1997	1996	1997
Likelihood of 'someone like me getting HIV (the AIDS virus)'	%	%	%	%
Very high	2	3	3	2
Quite high	8	6	5	4
Low	55	58	57	60
No risk	30	28	31	30
Don't know	6	5	5	4
Base = 100%	1399	990	1738	1230

Table 6.7 Respondents' assessment of the likelihood of 'someone like me getting another sexually transmitted disease' by year and sex
Adults aged 16-54 in 1996

	Men		Women	
	1996-1997			
Year	1996	1997	1996	1997
Likelihood of 'someone like me getting another sexually transmitted disease'	%	%	%	%
Very high	2	2	2	1
Quite high	7	5	5	4
Low	53	59	56	60
No risk	33	30	34	32
Don't know	5	3	4	3
Base = 100%	1399	990	1738	1230

Table 6.8 Whether would find it difficult to raise the subject of using a condom with a new partner by year and sex
Adults aged 16-54 in 1996

	Men		Women	
	1996-1997			
Year	1996	1997	1996	1997
Whether would find it difficult to raise the subject of using a condom	%	%	%	%
Strongly agree	6	5	7	7
Agree	10	8	12	9
Neither agree nor disagree	19	21	13	15
Disagree	47	49	45	47
Strongly disagree	18	17	23	22
Base = 100%	1388	988	1720	1227

Table 6.9 Whether would use a condom if 'in the near future they did have sex with a new partner' by year and sex
Adults aged 16-54 in 1996

	Men		Women	
	1996-1997			
Year	1996	1997	1996	1997
Whether would use a condom with a new partner	%	%	%	%
Would always use a condom	58	57	67	67
It would depend	31	34	17	17
Would never use a condom	1	2	1	1
Wouldn't contemplate having sex	10	7	15	14
Base = 100%	1392	987	1729	1229

Table 6.10 Whether reported a new partner in the last 12 months in 1997 by whether reported a new partner in the last 12 months in 1996 and sex
Adults aged 16-54 in 1996

Whether reported a new partner in the last 12 months in 1996	New partner	No new partner	No partner	Total
Whether reported a new partner in the last 12 months in 1997	%	%	%	%
Men				
New partner	56	8	25	20
No new partner	35	89	14	66
No partner	9	3	61	13
Base = 100%	*186*	*608*	*139*	*933*
Women				
New partner	50	7	17	15
No new partner	41	90	12	72
No partner	8	4	71	12
Base = 100%	*184*	*843*	*157*	*1184*

Table 6.11 Percentage using a condom with a new partner by year and sex
Adults aged 16-54 in 1996, reporting a new partner in the last year

Year	Men	Women	Men	Women
	Percentage using a condom with a new partner		Base = 100%	
1996	60	63	*315*	*287*
1997	59	53	*187*	*180*

All Change?   The Health Education Monitoring Survey one year on

Table 7.1 Number of occasions of sunburn in the last 12 months by year and sex
Adults aged 16-74 in 1996

	Men		Women	
				1996-1997
Year	**1996**	**1997**	**1996**	**1997**
Self-reported general health	%	%	%	%
Sunburnt in last 12 months	29	26	23	20
Once	17	17	15	14
Twice	7	6	5	4
Three times	2	2	1	1
Four or more	2	2	2	1
Not sunburnt	71	74	77	80
Can't remember	0	0	0	0
Base = 100%	*2042*	*1524*	*2599*	*1920*

Table 7.2 Occasions on which respondents use suncream by year and sex
Adults aged 16-74 in 1996

	Men		Women	
				1996-1997
Year	**1996**	**1997**	**1996**	**1997**
Occasions on which respondents use suncream	%	%	%	%
Uses suncream	61	63	74	79
Sunbathing abroad	41	40	47	47
Outdoors abroad, but not sunbathing	27	30	35	39
Sunbathing in this country	32	32	49	51
Outdoors in this country doing something else	26	30	38	42
Does not use suncream	38	37	23	21
Never goes out in the sun	1	1	2	3
*Base = 100%**	*2041*	*1525*	*2600*	*1920*

* Totals add to more than 100 because respondents could have given more than one answer.

Table 7.3 Whether having a suntan is important by year and sex

Adults aged 16-74 in 1996

1996-1997

Year	Men		Women	
	1996	**1997**	**1996**	**1997**
Whether having a suntan is important	%	%	%	%
Important	20	20	31	30
Not important	80	80	69	70
Don't know	0	-	0	0
Base = 100%	*1799*	*1334*	*2347*	*1746*

Table 7.4 Number of occasions of sunburn in the last 12 months in 1996 and 1997 by sex

Adults aged 16-74 in 1996

Number of occasions of sunburn in 1996	Once	Twice	Three times	Four or more	Not sunburnt	Total*
Number of occasions of sunburn in 1997	%	%	%	%	%	%
Men						
Sunburnt in last 12 months						
Once	30	32	17	12	12	17
Twice	11	18	22	16	2	6
Three times	1	3	9	12	1	2
Four or more	1	4	6	17	0	1
Not sunburnt	56	43	46	44	83	74
Can't remember	-	0	-	-	-	0
Base = 100%	*246*	*96*	*31*	*33*	*1097*	*1504*
Women						
Sunburnt in last 12 months						
Once	34	29	[3]	[7]	10	14
Twice	4	15	[5]	[4]	2	4
Three times	2	2	[3]	[1]	0	1
Four or more	2	5	[1]	[6]	0	1
Not sunburnt	58	48	[7]	[8]	88	80
Can't remember	1	1	[1]	-	0	0
Base = 100%	*252*	*79*	*20*	*26*	*1537*	*1914*

* Total includes a small number of 'don't knows'.

All Change? The Health Education Monitoring Survey one year on

Table 7.5 Number of occasions of sunburn in the last 12 months in 1997 by whether used a suncream in 1996 and sex

Adults aged 16-74 in 1996

Whether used a suncream in 1996	Yes	No	Never go out in the sun	Total*
Number of occasions of sunburn in 1997	%	%	%	%
Men				
Sunburnt in last 12 months				
Once	20	12	[1]	17
Twice	7	4	-	6
Three times	2	2	-	2
Four or more	2	1	-	1
Not sunburnt	70	80	[14]	74
Can't remember	0	0	-	6
Base = 100%	*906*	*583*	*15*	*1504*
Women				
Sunburnt in last 12 months				
Once	17	6	1	14
Twice	4	2	-	4
Three times	1	0	-	1
Four or more	1	1	-	1
Not sunburnt	76	90	99	80
Can't remember	0	0	-	0
Base = 100%	*1397*	*462*	*56*	*1915*

* Total includes a small number of 'don't knows'.

All Change? The Health Education Monitoring Survey one year on

69

Table 7.6 Number of occasions of sunburn in the last 12 months in 1997 by whether a suntan was important in 1996 and sex

Adults aged 16-74 in 1996

Whether a suntan was important in 1996	Very important	Fairly important	Not important	Total*
Number of occasions of sunburn in 1997	%	%	%	%
Men				
Sunburnt in last 12 months				
Once	26	18	17	18
Twice	7	9	6	6
Three times	-	1	2	2
Four or more	5	2	1	1
Not sunburnt	62	69	74	73
Can't remember	-	0	0	0
Base = 100%	*40*	*212*	*1079*	*1334*
Women				
Sunburnt in last 12 months				
Once	11	20	13	15
Twice	1	5	4	4
Three times	1	1	1	1
Four or more	2	1	1	1
Not sunburnt	84	72	82	79
Can't remember	-	0	0	0
Base = 100%	*82*	*421*	*1239*	*1748*

* Total includes a small number of 'don't knows'.

Table 7.7 Number of occasions of sunburn in the last 12 months in 1997 by whether agreed having a suntan is attractive in 1996 and sex
Adults aged 16-74 in 1996

Whether agreed that 'having a sun tan makes me look more attractive' in 1996	Strongly agreed	Agreed	Neither agreed nor disagreed	Disagreed	Strongly disagreed	Total
Number of occasions of sunburn in 1997	%	%	%	%	%	%
Men						
Sunburnt in last 12 months						
Once	[4]	20	20	13	22	18
Twice	[3]	7	7	4	3	6
Three times	[1]	2	2	1	2	2
Four or more	-	2	0	2	-	1
Not sunburnt	[14]	69	71	80	72	73
Can't remember	-	0	-	-	-	0
Base = 100%	*22*	*500*	*360*	*406*	*44*	*1332*
Women						
Sunburnt in last 12 months						
Once	14	17	17	11	11	15
Twice	3	3	3	5	8	4
Three times	1	1	1	1	-	1
Four or more	2	1	0	1	-	1
Not sunburnt	79	77	78	82	81	79
Can't remember	-	-	1	1	-	0
Base = 100%	*76*	*777*	*319*	*516*	*60*	*1748*

Table 7.8 Number of occasions of sunburn in the last 12 months in 1997 by whether agreed having a suntan makes me feel healthier in 1996 and sex
Adults aged 16-74 in 1996

Whether agreed that 'having a sun tan makes me feel healthier' in 1996	Strongly agreed	Agreed	Neither agreed nor disagreed	Disagreed	Strongly disagreed	Total
Number of occasions of sunburn in 1997	%	%	%	%	%	%
Men						
Sunburnt in last 12 months						
Once	17	21	16	15	16	18
Twice	10	7	4	5	15	6
Three times	-	1	2	2	4	2
Four or more	-	2	1	2	-	1
Not sunburnt	73	68	76	76	65	73
Can't remember	-	0	1	-	-	0
Base = 100%	*38*	*509*	*230*	*503*	*54*	*1334*
Women						
Sunburnt in last 12 months						
Once	14	17	17	11	10	15
Twice	3	4	3	3	7	4
Three times	2	1	1	1	1	1
Four or more	3	1	2	0	-	1
Not sunburnt	78	76	76	84	81	79
Can't remember	-	0	-	0	2	0
Base = 100%	*100*	*715*	*239*	*607*	*87*	*1748*

All Change? The Health Education Monitoring Survey one year on

Part C - *Reference Section*

Appendix A Sample design, response to the survey, weighting, characteristics of the responding sample and sampling errors

Introduction

This appendix gives details of the sample design used for the follow-up to the 1996 Health Education Monitoring Survey (HEMS), and of response to the survey. Although this report is part of the HEMS series, it is also designed to be used as an independent volume. This appendix therefore repeats the description of the 1996 sample which can also be found in the 1996 report. It also describes the weighting procedure applied to the data and presents information on the characteristics of the responding sample, on attrition between the original and follow-up interviews, and the sampling errors associated with the estimates shown in this report.

The sample design

The sample design for the 1996 survey was the same as that used for the 1995 survey; it followed the recommendations of a previous consultancy carried out by ONS for the Health Education Authority (HEA) in Summer 1994 which considered the optimum design for health surveys[1]. The review concluded that the Postcode Address File (PAF) is the most complete sampling frame available for general population surveys, and recommended that the sample design incorporate socio-economic as well as regional stratifiers.

A.2.1 Requirements of the sample

The selection process for the 1996 survey was designed to yield a representative sample of approximately 5,000 interviews with adults aged 16-74 living in private households in England. One person in this age-group was interviewed in each eligible household.

The sample was geographically clustered to give areas of a realistic size for interviewers to cover.

A.2.2 Selection of addresses and households

A sample of addresses was selected from the Postcode Address File (PAF). In order to select the appropriate number of addresses a stratified multi-stage random probability design was used. The stages in the selection of the sample were as follows:

(i)   The chosen primary sampling units (PSUs) were postcode sectors, which are similar in size to wards. Two hundred were selected by a systematic sampling method from a stratified list of postcode sectors. For this purpose all postcode sectors in England were stratified first by standard region, then according to the proportion of households in rented accommodation, then by the proportion of heads of household in socio-economic groups 1 to 5 and 13, i.e. professionals. Postcode sectors within the resulting strata were ranked by the proportion of households with a car. The regional stratification differentiated between metropolitan and non-metropolitan areas within standard regions. The other stratifying information was based on 1991 Census data.

(ii)   A random selection of postcode sectors was then made, with the chance of selection of each postcode sector being proportional to the total number of delivery points in the sector. From each of the 200 postcode sectors, 40 addresses were randomly selected, to give a total of 8,000 addresses.

A.2.3 Ineligible addresses

Since the requirement was for a sample of adults living in private households, business addresses and institutions were excluded at the sample selection stage as far as possible by using the PAF small users' file as the sampling frame. Twelve per cent (942) of the selected addresses did not contain a private household and were excluded from the set sample of addresses. These ineligible addresses included demolished or permanently empty addresses, addresses used only on an occasional basis and business premises and institutions where there was no resident private household.

A.2.4 Conversion of addresses to households

The PAF is a list of delivery points for mail so most households within multi-occupied addresses are separately listed on the frame. It is estimated, however, that a small proportion (less than 2%) of addresses on the PAF contain more than one private household.

Since each address listed on the PAF was given only one chance of selection for the HEMS sample, additional procedures were carried out in the field by interviewers at addresses found to contain more than one household in order to ensure that all households were given a chance of selection. Where the sampled address contained more than one private household, interviewers were asked to interview at all households up to a maximum of three. In the rare event that an address contained more than three households, the interviewer was instructed to list the households systematically and then three were chosen at random by reference to a selection table.

In order to limit workloads a maximum of four extra households per quota of addresses was allowed on this survey. In total, 94 extra households were identified in this way for inclusion in the survey, resulting in 7,152 households to be approached by interviewer. Twelve per cent (842) of these households contained no-one aged 16-74. Thus the total eligible sample of households was 6,310.

Sampling individuals within households

As noted above, one adult aged 16-74 was interviewed in each eligible household. This was done in preference to interviewing all eligible adults because it helped interviewers to carry out inter-views in private and obtain more reliable information. It also ensured that respondents' answers, particularly to the attitudinal questions, were not contaminated by hearing other household members' answers. Finally, individuals in households tend to be similar to one another and where households differ markedly from one another, the resultant clustering can lead to a substantial increase in the standard error around survey estimates. This is particularly true in a topic area such as health behaviours where household members may influence each other.

In households where there was more than one person aged 16-74, the interviewer selected one person at random for interview, ensuring that all household members in the eligible age range had the same chance of being selected.

The selection procedure carried out at the household was a standard Social Survey Division procedure and was as follows:

(i)   The interviewers listed everyone in the household on a selection sheet. They then numbered those aged 16 to 74 in order of age, eldest first.

(ii)   The person to be interviewed was then defined by reference to a selection table which was printed on a reference card.

(iii) The card indicated which one of the eligible people should be selected for a given address, depending upon the serial number of the address and the number of eligible people in the household.

The selection table was based on those designed by Kish, which gave a close approximation to the proper fractional representation of each eligible adult in the household for up to six adults[2]. For this survey, selection tables for up to 8 eligible adults were used and a different set of possible selections was shown for each of the 40 addresses in each postcode sector.

In theory this meant that in households with nine or more eligible people some people would not get a chance of selection. In practice no households as large as this were found on the survey.

Where the person who had been selected for interview was not the person who had given the interviewer the household details, interviewers made arrangements to interview the selected person.

In 1996, the response rate for the face-to-face interviews was 74%. An additional 2% (145 cases) were interviewed by proxy.

The sample for the 1997 survey

At the end of the 1996 interview, respondents were asked whether they would be willing to participate in any follow-up interviews. At this stage, 4424 agreed in principle, and gave the interviewer usable details of how they could be contacted in the future. A 'keeping-in-touch' (KITE) letter was sent to those respondents in January 1997, saying that we hoped to interview them again in Summer 1997. A form listing their details was enclosed with the letter, which they were asked to amend and return if any of the details were incorrect. At this stage, a small proportion of respondents wrote to say they were unwilling to take part in the follow-up interview, and some letters were returned by the Post Office as 'address unknown'. The number of addresses issued to interviewers for the 1997 survey was 4,314. (**Tables A.1-A.2**)

An advance letter was sent to all 4,314 respondents just before the start of fieldwork. The letter was shorter than in previous years; being redesigned in line with the findings of methodological work carried out by SSD on advance letters[3].

A proportion of respondents had moved house between the two waves of the survey. Where a forwarding address was known, movers were interviewed at their new address by the HEMS interviewer working in the area. Where no HEMS interviewer was available, the interview was carried out on the telephone by SSD's Telephone Unit. In total, 116 respondents were interviewed on the telephone, including 10 respondents interviewed by proxy. Those interviewed on the telephone were not asked the questions in the self-completion module.

Response to the survey

Table A.2 shows the outcome in 1997 for the sample of eligible individuals. Eighty per cent of adults agreed to take part in the survey. An additional 1% of eligible individuals were interviewed by proxy. Ten per cent refused to take part, either in response to the KITE letter (1%), before the interviewer visited the address (1%), or at the main interview stage (8%). Interviewers were unable to contact 9% of respondents: in approximately 4% of cases, respondents were known to have moved since being interviewed in 1996 but left no forwarding address. Ten respond-ents were unable to be interviewed, either in person or by proxy, because they were too ill or absent for the whole field period, or because of language difficulties. Including those who refused any follow-up visit at the end of the 1996 interview, the total attrition between 1996 and 1997 was 27%. (**Table A.2**)

Adults aged 16-55 who were interviewed face-to-face were eligible for the self-completion module on drugs and sexual health. A small number (2) had terminated the interview before reaching this module. The overwhelming majority (99%) of eligible respondents agreed to take part in the self-completion. Eighty seven per cent recorded their own answers on the laptop, while 8% asked the interviewer to key their answers in for them. Three respondents completed the drugs section but refused the sexual health section and four completed the sexual health section but refused to answer questions on the drugs section. (**Table A.3**)

Non-response and weighting

Reweighting procedures were used to compensate for differing probabilities of selection and non-response bias in the sample. The final weights for the 1997 sample were a combination of the 1996 weights and a weight which took account of attrition between the two years of the survey.

A.6.1. Weighting applied to the 1996 survey

In 1996, there were two steps to the weighting. Firstly, weights were applied to take account of the different probabilities of selecting respondents in differently sized households. Secondly, all respondents were given a weight to represent the age-sex-region structure of the total national population of England living in private households.

A.6.1.1 Weighting for probability of selection

Sample weights to allow for the different probabilities of selecting a respondent in differently sized households corresponded to the number of members of the household aged 16-74. Thus, an adult in a single-person household was given a weight of one, while a respondent in a household with three people aged 16-74 was given a weight of three.

A.6.1.2 Weighting for non-response bias

As mentioned, the response rate for the face-to-face interviews was 74% in 1996. An additional 2% (145 cases) were interviewed by proxy. A weight for non-response was applied to the full and partial interviews only as only these cases were used for analysis. The cases where interviews were carried out by proxy were therefore given a weight of one for non-response so that in effect they were only re-weighted for probability of selection.

The age, sex, regional, marital status and ethnic origin distributions of the responding sample on the 1996 HEMS were compared with other national estimates, having first been reweighted for household size.

Estimates of age, sex, region and ethnic origin were taken from the December 1995 to February 1996 quarter of the Labour Force Survey (LFS) for England only. The LFS is a large sample survey carried out quarterly; the data are weighted and grossed to represent the total population. The 1995 mid-year population estimates which are based on the 1991 Census were also looked at but because these estimates include individuals living in institutions it was decided that the LFS estimates were more appropriate for comparison with HEMS. Estimates for marital status were taken from the 1994 General Household Survey (GHS)[4] as the categories for marital status used by the LFS differ from those used by HEMS. HEMS and the GHS use the same categories.

The HEMS sample under-represented men as a whole, although among men the age breakdown was similar to the LFS. The HEMS sample under-represented women aged 16-19 and over-represented women aged 40-44. The sample also under-represented people, particularly women, living in Greater London. (Tables A.4-A.5)

There were no significant differences between the proportions of GHS and HEMS respondents in different marital statuses. It should be noted that although the GHS results are themselves estimates and therefore subject to bias, Foster et al[5] concluded that evidence from the 1991 Census-linked study of the GHS sample showed that the non-response bias was relatively modest. (Table A.6)

With regard to ethnic origin the HEMS sample slightly under-represented Bangladeshi women. It was decided not to re-weight for this, however, as the numbers were too small to use for weighting and ethnic origin was not used in the analysis. (Table A.7)

The 1996 HEMS sample was therefore reweighted to give the correct proportions for age, sex and region. When the number of men and women living in London was broken down by age the numbers in some of the cells were too small to use for weighting so a new regional variable; distinguishing between those living in the South East and those not living in the South East was created and used for weighting. The age-sex-region weights were produced by dividing the population proportion by the sample proportion. The weights are shown in Table A.8. Categories with weights of less than 1.0 were over-represented in the HEMS responding sample and those with weights of more than 1.0 were under-represented. (Table A.8)

A.6.1.3 Creating a final weight in 1996

The final weight applied to the 1996 sample was the product of these two sets of weights. For example, applying the product of the two weights would give a weight of 3.87 for a female aged 16-24 living in the South East in a household containing three eligible people (1.29 x 3).

A.6.2 Creating a weight in 1997

Respondents and non-respondents to the 1997 survey were compared on a number of socio-demographic and other variables, using data from the 1996 survey, and the results are shown in Tables A.9-A.10. These show that equal proportions of men and women responded in 1997, but that younger respondents, those living in London and those classified as belonging to Social Classes IV and V, or who had never worked, belonged to the Armed Forces or whose occupation was unclassified in 1996 had lower response rates than other groups of informants. (Tables A.9-A.10)

Differences between responders and non-responders were modelled using An SPSS package called CHAID (Chi-squared automatic interaction detector). CHAID performs segmentational modelling, which divides a population into two or more distinct groups based on categories of the 'best' predictor of a dependent variable. It then splits each of these groups into smaller sub-groups based on other predictor variables. The segments which CHAID derives are mutually exclusive and exhaustive; that is, the segments do not overlap and each case is contained in exactly one segment[6]. The segments are then used as weighting classes.

The dependent variable for the analysis was response/non-response to the 1997 survey. Several models were run using data from the 1996 survey; the final one chosen used age, region, social class, marital status, cigarette smoking status, whether respondents had a limiting, non-limiting or no long-standing illness, frequency of participation in at least moderate-intensity physical activity, and whether or not respondents had been sunburnt in the 12 months before interview as predictor variables. All but the last two were significant.

All Change? The Health Education Monitoring Survey one year on

75

Age was the most important predictor of response; attrition among those aged 16-34 in 1996 was 26.9%, compared with a rate of 15.2% among the 35-74 age-group. Among those aged 16-34, the next most important predictor was region while, for those aged 35-74 it was social class. The lowest level of attrition was among respondents aged 35-74 who belonged to Social Class III (Manual) and who reported a long-standing illness in 1996; the response rate for this group was 89%. The highest attrition was among respondents aged 16-34 who were members of the Armed Forces or who had never worked, and who were resident in Greater London, the Outer Metropolitan area or the South West; their response rate in 1997 was 52%. The weight for each of these groups was calculated by dividing the overall response rate by the response rate for that segment. The resulting segments, or groups, together with the proportions in each and the associated weights, are shown in **Table A.11**.

The pattern of attrition between the two waves of the survey is very similar to that observed between the two waves of the Health and Lifestyles Survey (HALS1 and HALS2)[7]. Attrition in that survey was highest among those aged 18-34, as for HEMS, those living in London and urban areas in general. Other variables associated with attrition for HALS were being non-white, a private renter, single, living in a single-person household, not being in the labour force, having no qualifications and having a low income. Again, as for HEMS, attrition was linked to some non-demographic variables; it was higher among regular smokers (although the main cause of attrition among this group was death, whereas HEMS smokers in the 16-34 age-group were most likely not to be interviewed at the second wave), and among those reporting no long-standing illness. The general conclusion drawn by the researchers was that a person's own position on a series of health-related variables does not consciously affect their decision to participate in a health survey.

For both HEMS and HALS, there was some similarity between the characteristics of non-responders in Waves 1 and 2; the young and those living in London and the South East were more likely to be non-responders for HEMS in 1996 and 1997.

A final weight for 1997 was created by multiplying the final 1996 weight by the weight derived from the CHAID analysis.

The tables in the main body of the report present weighted proportions, and unweighted bases.

The accuracy of the survey results

Like all estimates based on samples, the results of the HEMS survey are subject to variations and errors. The total error associated with any survey estimate is the difference between the estimate derived from the data collected and the true value for the population. The total error can be divided into two main types of error: systematic error and random error.

Systematic error is often referred to as bias. Bias can arise because the sampling frame is incomplete, because of variation in the way interviewers ask questions and record answers, or because non-respondents to the survey have different characteristics to respondents. When designing surveys considerable effort is made to minimise systematic error; these include training interviewers to maximise response rates and to ask questions in a standard way, and carrying out pilot work to test questions and survey procedures and to assess whether the interview and individual questions are

understood by and acceptable to respondents. Nonetheless, some systematic error is likely to remain.

Random error occurs because survey estimates are based not on the whole population but only a sample of it. There may be chance variations between such a sample and the whole population. If a number of repeats of the same survey were carried out, this error could be expected to average to zero. The sampling variations depend on both the size of the sample and its design.

Statistical theory, however, enables estimates to be made of how close the survey results are to the true population values for each characteristic. A statistical measure of variation, the standard error, can be estimated from the values obtained for the sample, and provides a measure of the statistical precision of the survey estimate. This allows confidence intervals to be calculated around the sample estimate which give an indication of the range in which the true population value is likely to fall. The confidence interval generally used in survey research is the 95% confidence interval; it comprises the range of values from two standard errors below the estimate to two standard errors above the estimate.

For results based on simple random samples, without clustering or stratification, the estimation of standard errors is straightforward. When, as in the case of the HEMS and most other surveys, the sample design is not a simple random sample, a more complex calculation, using a formula which takes account of the random variation of the denominator and the stratification and clustering of the sample design, is necessary[8]. Stratification tends to reduce the standard error, while clustering tends to increase it.

In a complex sample design, the size of the standard error depends on how the characteristic of interest is spread within and between primary sampling units and between strata. So, for example, characteristics likely to be associated with the primary sampling unit, postcode sectors, will tend to have larger standard errors.

Tables A.12-A.20 show the standard error and 95% confidence intervals for selected survey estimates. They also show the design factor, or deft; the ratio of the standard error to the standard error that would have resulted had the survey design been a simple random sample of the same size. This is often used to give a broad indication of the degree of clustering. The tables do not cover all the topics discussed in the report; where possible, standard errors were calculated for a different set of estimates from those used in 1995 and 1996.

Design factors of less than 1.2 are considered to be small and indicate that the characteristic is not markedly clustered. However, substantial design factors of 1.2 or more were recorded for a number of characteristics, and this is reflected in being able to make less precise estimates for these characteristics than for other survey measures. A higher design factor indicates that the characteristic is more clustered geographically.

Among the sample characteristics covered in Table A.12, design factors of 1.2 or higher were found for the youngest age-groups, highest qualification level and for married, cohabiting and single men , and for cohabiting and single women. The design factors were also high for men in all social classes except Social Class I and II. For the health and health-related behaviour variables, with the exception of men's opinions of the safety of drugs, and respondents' assessment of whether they had changed their diet in the last year, most of the occurrences of design factors of 1.2 or more were for single categories of a variable of interest. (**Tables A.12-A.20**)

Notes and references

1. Elliot D. *Optimising sample designs for surveys of health and related behaviour and attitudes.* in *Survey Methodology Bulletin*, Vol. 36, 1995, pp. 8-17.

2. Kish L. *Survey Sampling.* J Wiley & Sons Ltd (London 1965).

3. White A and Freeth S. Improving advance letters, in *Survey Methodology Bulletin*, Vol. 40, 1997, pp. 23-28.

4. The data from the 1995 GHS were not available at the time the HEMS weighting was carried out.

5. Foster K et al. *General Household Survey 1993.* HMSO (London 1995).

6. Magidson, J. *SPSS for Windows CHAID.* Statistical Innovations Inc. (1993)

7. Gray R et al. Exploring survey non-response: the effect of attrition on a follow-up of the 1984-5 health and lifestyle survey, in *The Statistician,* vol. 45, 2, 1996, pp. 163-183.

8. For a full description of the method used to calculate standard errors for complex survey design, see Butcher B and Elliot D. A Sampling Errors Manual. HMSO (London 1992).

All Change? The Health Education Monitoring Survey one year on

77

Table A.1 The sample of respondents from the 1996 survey

	No.
Responded to 1996 survey	4790
Did not agree to recall	366
Selected respondents	4424
Ineligible respondents	110
Respondent had moved outside England	31
Respondent had died	22
Respondent had been institutionalised	6
Demolished, derelict, returned by Post Office	51
Total eligible sample of respondents for 1997	4314

Table A.3 Response of adults aged 16-55 to the self-completion module

Response	No.	%
Adults aged 16-55	2349	100
Telephone interview	90	4
Eligible for self-completion	2259	96
Co-operated with self-completion	2228	95
Completed drugs section only	*3*	*0*
Completed sexual health section only	*4*	*0*
Completed by respondent	*2053*	*87*
Completed by interviewer	*175*	*8*
Self-completion refused	29	1
Did not complete main interview	2	0

Table A.2 Response of adults to follow-up interview

Response	No.	%
Set sample of respondents	4314	100
Fully co-operating adults	3451	80
Partially co-operating adults	4	0
Proxy interview carried out	34	1
Non-responding adults	825	19
Refusal	437	10
refusal to KITE letter	*41*	*1*
direct to HQ	*36*	*1*
by sampled person	*360*	*8*
Non-contact	378	9
moved, no forwarding address	*178*	*4*
moved within England, unable to contact	*23*	*1*
other unable to contact	*177*	*4*
No proxy interview possible	10	0

Table A.4 Distribution of responders to 1996 HEMS compared to Labour Force Survey (LFS) estimates for England by age and sex

Age group	Men HEMS* %	Men LFS† %	Women HEMS* %	Women LFS† %	All HEMS* %	All LFS† %
16-19	7.0	6.5	4.5	6.1	5.6	6.3
20-24	8.6	9.1	8.4	8.6	8.5	8.9
25-29	9.9	11.1	10.5	10.6	10.2	10.9
30-34	10.4	11.7	11.1	11.2	10.8	11.4
35-39	10.1	10.1	10.5	9.9	10.3	10.0
40-44	8.5	9.1	11.1	9.0	9.9	9.0
45-49	10.2	9.9	8.7	9.8	9.4	9.8
50-54	8.0	8.1	8.7	8.1	8.3	8.1
55-59	7.6	7.1	6.9	7.1	7.2	7.1
60-64	7.0	6.4	6.2	6.6	6.6	6.5
65-69	6.8	5.9	7.1	6.6	7.0	6.2
70-74	6.0	5.1	6.3	6.4	6.1	5.7
Base = 100%	2,044	17,393,607	2,601	17,500,137	4,645	34,893,744

* HEMS proportions are reweighted for number of adults in household.

† LFS survey estimates are weighted and grossed to the population estimates for England.

Table A.5 Distribution of responders to 1996 HEMS compared to Labour Force Survey (LFS) estimates for England by standard region

Standard region	Men HEMS* %	Men LFS† %	Women HEMS* %	Women LFS† %	All HEMS* %	All LFS† %
North	5.8	6.3	6.8	6.4	6.4	6.4
Yorkshire and Humberside	11.1	10.4	11.7	10.3	11.4	10.4
North West	13.2	13.0	13.9	13.1	13.6	13.0
East Midlands	9.2	8.5	9.2	8.5	9.2	8.5
West Midlands	10.5	10.9	11.2	10.8	10.9	10.9
East Anglia	4.1	4.4	4.8	4.4	4.5	4.4
Greater London	12.6	14.4	11.7	14.5	12.1	14.4
South East	22.8	22.3	21.3	22.3	22.0	22.3
South West	10.7	9.8	9.3	9.8	9.9	9.8
Base = 100%	2,044	17,393,607	2,601	17,500,137	4,645	34,893,744

* HEMS proportions are reweighted for number of adults in household.

† LFS survey estimates are weighted and grossed to the population estimates for England.

Table A.6 Distribution of responders to 1996 HEMS compared to GHS 1994 by marital status

	Men		Women		All	
	HEMS*	GHS 1994	HEMS*	GHS 1994	HEMS*	GHS 1994
Marital status	%	%	%	%	%	%
Married	59.5	60.5	58.0	57.3	58.7	58.9
Cohabiting	7.6	7.5	8.1	7.4	7.9	7.4
Single	25.0	24.5	18.5	19.1	21.5	21.7
Widowed	2.4	2.3	7.1	7.4	4.9	5.0
Divorced	3.9	3.8	5.8	6.3	4.9	5.1
Separated	1.3	1.3	2.5	2.5	2.0	1.9
Base = 100%	*2044*	*6946*	*2601*	*7433*	*4645*	*14379*

* HEMS proportions are reweighted for number of adults in household.

Table A.7 Distribution of responders to 1996 HEMS compared to Labour Force Survey by ethnic origin and sex

	Men		Women		All	
	HEMS*	LFS†	HEMS*	LFS†	HEMS*	LFS†
Ethnic Origin	%	%	%	%	%	%
White	94.4	93.9	94.7	94.0	94.5	94.0
Indian	1.1	1.8	1.2	1.7	1.4	1.7
Pakistani	0.7	0.9	0.5	0.9	0.6	0.9
Bangladeshi	0.5	0.4	0.1	0.3	0.3	0.3
Black- Caribbean	0.6	0.9	1.2	1.1	0.9	1.0
Other ethnic group	2.7	2.0	1.9	2.0	2.2	2.0
Base	*2,043*	*17,388,346*	*2,043*	*17,496,583*	*4,640*	*34,884,930*

* HEMS proportions are reweighted for number of adults in household.
† LFS survey estimates are weighted and grossed to the population estimates for England.

All Change? The Health Education Monitoring Survey one year on

Table A.8 1996 age-sex-region weights

	LFS population totals	LFS proportion	Total responding in sample	Sample proportion	Age-sex-region weight
South East					
Men					
16-24	986922	2.8	84	2.7	1.04
25-39	2234842	6.4	256	5.3	1.21
40-54	1711435	4.9	193	4.3	1.14
55-74	1469791	4.2	191	3.9	1.08
Women					
16-24	949075	2.7	76	2.1	1.29
25-39	2170318	6.2	307	6.2	1.00
40-54	1726800	4.9	218	5.1	0.97
55-74	1607741	4.6	262	4.5	1.02
Not South East					
Men					
16-24	1761543	5.0	140	4.4	1.14
25-39	3501364	10.0	399	8.6	1.16
40-45	3002100	8.6	353	7.9	1.09
55-74	2779219	7.9	428	8.6	0.92
Women					
16-24	1664237	4.8	190	4.9	0.97
25-39	3384445	9.7	558	11.2	0.86
40-54	2991626	8.5	429	10.3	0.83
55-74	3049249	8.7	561	9.9	0.88
Base = 100%	*34990707*	*100*	*4645*	*100*	

Table A.9 Characteristics of responders and non-responders to the 1997 survey
Adults responding to the 1996 survey

Estimate		Responders in 1997	Non-responders in 1997	Did not agree to follow-up interview in 1996	Bases = 100%
		Percentage			
Sex					
Male	%	72	18	9	2138
Female	%	73	17	10	2652
Age					
16-24	%	62	27	11	509
25-34	%	67	22	11	1059
35-44	%	78	14	8	963
45-54	%	77	15	9	788
55-64	%	76	14	9	686
65-74	%	75	14	11	785
Standard region					
North	%	78	11	10	315
Yorkshire and Humberside	%	69	18	14	540
North West	%	71	21	8	652
East Midlands	%	76	18	6	426
West Midlands	%	73	17	10	514
East Anglia	%	74	15	12	212
Greater London	%	65	21	14	623
Outer Metropolitan and Outer South East	%	75	16	8	1028
South West	%	77	16	7	480
Marital status					
Single	%	65	24	12	1041
Married, cohabiting	%	75	16	9	2861
Widowed, divorced or separated	%	76	15	9	888
Social class					
I & II	%	76	15	9	1509
III (NM)	%	75	16	9	1071
III (M)	%	75	17	8	808
IV & V	%	68	20	12	1078
Unclassified*	%	59	25	16	321

* Members of the Armed Forces, persons in inadequately described occupations and persons who have never worked.

Table A.10 Selected estimates for responders and non-responders to the 1997 survey
Adults responding to the 1996 survey

Estimate		Responders in 1997	Non-responders in 1997	Did not agree to follow-up interview in 1996	Bases = 100%
			Percentage		
Cigarette smoking status					
Smoked 20+ cigarettes per day	%	70	23	7	445
10-19 cigarettes a day	%	68	24	8	552
0-9 cigarettes a day	%	75	18	7	400
No of cigarettes not known	%	[5]	[3]	-	8
Ex regular smoker	%	77	14	8	1137
Never smoked regularly	%	75	16	9	2100
Alcohol consumption in units per week					
Men					
Non-drinker	%	73	15	11	123
Under one	%	78	14	8	146
1-10	%	74	19	7	631
11-21	%	75	19	6	489
22-35	%	77	17	6	337
35-50	%	75	22	3	148
51 or over	%	65	22	14	133
Women					
Non-drinker	%	71	17	12	278
Under one	%	71	18	11	472
1-7	%	77	15	8	994
8-14	%	75	15	10	422
15-25	%	76	19	5	246
26-35	%	68	26	7	74
36 or over	%	65	32	3	74
Number of occasions of at least moderate activity per week					
0-3	%	73	16	11	1222
4-11	%	76	16	8	1246
12-19	%	75	18	7	601
20 or more	%	74	20	6	1573
Whether sunburnt in the last 12 months					
Yes	%	72	20	7	1103
No	%	75	17	8	3533
Can't remember	%	[1]	[2]	[3]	6
Frequency of consumption of bread, fruit, vegetables or salad and potatoes, pasta or rice					
Ate foods from all three groups daily	%	77	14	9	1760
Frequency of eating foods from all three groups varied	%	73	20	8	2855
Ate foods from all three groups 1-2 times a week	%	[18]	[7]	-	25
Type of fats eaten					
Ate foods high in saturated fats	%	[18]	[4]	[4]	26
Saturated fat content varied	%	74	18	8	3372
Ate foods low in saturated fats	%	76	17	7	1010
Whether reported a long-standing illness					
Limiting long-standing illness	%	76	15	9	988
Non-limiting long-standing illness	%	78	16	7	769
No long-standing illness	%	73	19	8	2884

Table A.11 1997 weighting classes

Class	Weighting class	No.*	%	Response rate	Weight
				Adults participating in a face-to-face interview in the 1996 survey	
	Aged 16-34				
	Regions I-VI				
1	Single	819	9.9	73.5	1.096
2	Married or cohabiting, widowed, divorced or separated	788	9.6	80.6	0.999
	Regions V11-IX				
	Social Classes I-IV				
2	Smokes 10+ cigarettes per day	284	3.4	60.1	1.340
4	Smokes less than 10 or non-smoker, aged 16-24	380	4.6	68.1	1.182
5	Smokes less than 10 or non-smoker, aged 25-34	577	7.0	77.8	1.035
6	Armed forces, never worked	160	1.9	52.4	1.538
	Aged 35-74				
7	Social Classes I-III (N-M)	2909	35.3	87.7	0.918
	Social Class III (M)				
8	Has a long-standing illness	439	5.3	88.9	0.906
9	Has no long-standing illness	556	6.7	80.3	1.003
	Social Classes IV and V				
	Regions I-VII				
	Has a long-standing illness				
10	Married, cohabiting or single	368	4.5	83.8	0.961
11	Divorced, widowed or separated	82	1.0	67.7	1.189
12	Has no long-standing illness	488	5.9	73.2	1.100
13	Region VIII	279	3.4	86.6	0.909
14	Region IX	121	1.5	72.4	1.112
	All		8250	100	80.5

* Weighted sample size

All Change? The Health Education Monitoring Survey one year on

Table A.12 Standard errors and 95% confidence intervals for socio-demographic variables

Base	Characteristic	%(p)	Sample size	Standard error of p	95% confidence interval	Deft
	Age					
Men	16-24	14.7	1525	1.31	12.1 – 17.3	1.45
	25-34	19.4	1525	1.23	17.0 – 21.8	1.21
	35-44	21.7	1525	1.12	19.5 – 23.9	1.06
	45-54	19.0	1525	1.10	16.8 – 21.2	1.09
	55-64	12.6	1525	0.81	11.0 – 14.2	0.95
	65-74	12.6	1525	0.89	10.9 – 14.3	1.05
Women	16-24	11.8	1923	1.01	9.8 – 13.8	1.37
	25-34	21.7	1923	1.11	19.5 – 23.9	1.18
	35-44	22.5	1923	1.09	20.4 – 24.6	1.15
	45-54	16.9	1923	0.97	15.0 – 18.8	1.13
	55-64	13.3	1923	0.91	11.5 – 15.1	1.18
	65-74	13.8	1923	0.79	12.3 – 15.3	1.01
	Social class of respondent					
Men	I and II	37.7	1525	1.45	34.9 – 40.5	1.17
(excluding armed	III Non-Manual	11.2	1525	1.03	9.2 – 13.2	1.27
forces, never worked	III Manual	27.8	1525	1.56	24.7 – 30.9	1.36
and not known)	IV and V	19.4	1525	1.30	16.9 – 21.9	1.28
Women	I and II	27.4	1923	1.12	25.2 – 29.6	1.10
(excluding armed	III Non-Manual	35.1	1923	1.22	32.7 – 37.5	1.12
forces, never worked	III Manual	8.0	1923	0.68	6.6 – 9.3	1.10
and not known)	IV and V	25.3	1923	1.20	22.9 – 27.7	1.21
	Highest qualification level					
Men	'A' level or above	39.6	1524	1.62	36.4 – 42.8	1.29
	Other qualifications	38.5	1524	1.57	35.4 – 41.6	1.26
	No qualifications	21.9	1524	1.36	19.2 – 24.6	1.28
Women	'A' level or above	30.9	1922	1.39	28.3 – 33.6	1.32
	Other qualifications	40.7	1922	1.34	38.1 – 43.3	1.19
	No qualifications	28.4	1922	1.26	26.0 – 30.9	1.22
	Marital status					
Men	Married	60.8	1525	1.57	57.7 – 63.9	1.25
	Cohabiting	7.4	1525	0.83	5.8 – 9.0	1.23
	Single	24.2	1525	1.42	21.4 – 27.0	1.30
	Widowed/separated/divorced	7.6	1525	0.59	6.4 – 8.7	0.88
Women	Married	56.9	1923	1.35	54.3 – 59.5	1.19
	Cohabiting	8.3	1923	0.79	6.8 – 9.9	1.25
	Single	18.4	1923	1.11	16.2 – 20.5	1.26
	Widowed/separated/divorced	16.4	1923	0.78	14.9 – 17.9	0.93

Table A.13 Standard errors and 95% confidence intervals for general health variables

Base	Characteristic	%(p)	Sample size	Standard error of p	95% confidence interval	Deft
	Level of self-reported stress					
Men	No, small stress	42.6	1524	1.45	39.8 – 45.4	1.14
	Moderate or large stress	57.4	1524	1.45	54.6 – 60.2	1.14
Women	No, small stress	31.8	1922	1.25	29.4 – 34.3	1.17
	Moderate or large stress	68.2	1922	1.25	65.8 – 70.7	1.18

Table A.14 Standard errors and 95% confidence intervals for smoking variables

Base	Characteristic	%(p)	Sample size	Standard error of p	95% confidence interval	Deft
	Cigarette smoking status					
Men	Heavy smoker	10.6	1516	0.77	9.1 – 12.1	0.97
	Moderate smoker	11.5	1516	1.01	9.5 – 13.5	1.24
	Light smoker	7.8	1516	0.79	6.3 – 9.3	1.15
	Ex-regular smoker	27.4	1516	1.29	24.9 – 29.9	1.12
	Never smoked regularly	42.4	1516	1.41	39.6 – 45.2	1.11
Women	Heavy smoker	6.9	1919	0.65	5.6 – 8.2	1.13
	Moderate smoker	11.9	1919	0.88	10.2 – 13.6	1.18
	Light smoker	9.8	1919	0.82	8.2 – 11.4	1.20
	Ex-regular smoker	19.2	1919	1.02	17.2 – 21.2	1.13
	Never smoked regularly	52.2	1919	1.41	49.4 – 55.0	1.24
	Whether thinks level of smoking is different to a year ago					
Men: smokers	Smoking more	11.8	444	1.69	8.5 – 15.1	1.10
	Smoking about same	50.9	444	2.59	45.8 – 56.0	1.09
	Smoking less	34.4	444	2.58	29.3 – 39.5	1.14
	Didn't smoke regularly	2.9	444	1.11	0.7 – 5.1	1.38
Women: smokers	Smoking more	16.0	548	1.73	12.6 – 19.4	1.10
	Smoking about same	49.3	548	2.23	44.9 – 53.7	1.04
	Smoking less	32.7	548	2.22	28.3 – 37.1	1.11
	Didn't smoke regularly	2.0	548	0.60	0.8 – 3.2	1.01

Table A.15 Standard errors and 95% confidence intervals for drinking variables

Base	Characteristic	%(p)	Sample size	Standard error of p	95% confidence interval	Deft
	Current alcohol consumption (units per week)					
Men	None, less than one unit	12.1	1517	1.02	10.1 – 14.1	1.22
	1-21 units	57.6	1517	1.43	54.8 – 60.4	1.13
	22-50 units	24.0	1517	1.20	21.6 – 26.4	1.10
	51 or more units	6.3	1517	0.64	5.0 – 7.6	1.03
Women	None, less than one unit	25.5	1921	1.09	23.4 – 27.6	1.10
	1-14 units	57.6	1921	1.21	55.2 – 60.0	1.07
	15-35 units	14.2	1921	0.98	12.3 – 16.1	1.23
	36 or more units	2.7	1921	0.46	1.8 – 3.6	1.24
	Whether thinks drinking is different to a year ago					
Men	Drinking more	13.1	1443	1.11	10.9 – 15.3	1.25
	Drinking about same	61.5	1443	1.51	58.5 – 64.5	1.18
	Drinking less	25.4	1443	1.47	22.5 – 28.3	1.29
Women	Drinking more	11.8	1727	0.92	10.0 – 13.6	1.19
	Drinking about same	62.2	1727	1.34	59.6 – 64.8	1.15
	Drinking less	26.0	1727	1.12	23.8 – 28.2	1.06

All Change? The Health Education Monitoring Survey one year on

87

Table A.16 Standard errors and 95% confidence intervals for drugs variables

Base	Characteristic	%(p)	Sample size	Standard error of p	95% confidence interval	Deft
	Whether had ever used any drug					
Men		38.6	991	1.72	35.2 – 42.0	1.11
Women		27.3	1229	1.51	24.3 – 30.3	1.19
	Whether had used any drug in the last year					
Men		15.4	991	1.23	13.0 – 17.8	1.07
Women		10.8	1229	0.99	8.9 – 12.7	1.11
	Whether had used any drug in the last month					
Men		10.4	991	1.11	8.2 – 12.6	1.14
Women		6.5	1229	0.79	5.0 – 8.1	1.13
	Whether agrees that 'I don't mind other people using drugs'					
Men	Agree	24.3	990	1.51	21.3 – 27.3	1.11
	Disagree	48.0	990	1.83	44.4 – 51.6	1.15
	Neither agree nor disagree	27.6	990	1.68	24.3 – 30.9	1.18
Women	Agree	17.8	1229	1.20	15.4 – 20.2	1.10
	Disagree	54.2	1229	1.76	50.8 – 57.6	1.24
	Neither agree nor disagree	28.0	1229	1.51	25.0 – 31.0	1.18
	Whether drugs are safe to use or not					
Men	All drugs are safe to use (as long as you know what you're doing)	1.8	989	0.54	0.7 – 2.9	1.25
	Some drugs are safe to use (as long as you know what you're doing)	30.2	989	1.84	26.6 – 33.8	1.26
	No drugs are safe to use	57.4	989	1.91	53.7 – 61.1	1.22
	I don't know whether drugs are safe to use or not	10.6	989	0.99	8.7 – 12.5	1.01
Women	All drugs are safe to use (as long as you know what you're doing)	0.9	1229	0.31	0.3 – 1.5	1.15
	Some drugs are safe to use (as long as you know what you're doing)	21.8	1229	1.40	19.1 – 24.5	1.19
	No drugs are safe to use	68.0	1229	1.51	65.0 – 71.0	1.13
	I don't know whether drugs are safe to use or not	9.3	1229	0.83	7.7 – 10.9	1.00

Table A.17 Standard errors and 95% confidence intervals for physical activity variables

Base	Characteristic	%(p)	Sample size	Standard error of p	95% confidence interval	Deft
	Whether thinks level of activity is different to a year ago					
Men	More active	21.2	1484	1.27	18.7 – 23.7	1.20
	About as active	56.9	1484	1.42	54.1 – 59.7	1.10
	Less active	21.9	1484	1.27	19.4 – 24.4	1.18
Women	More active	26.9	1868	1.22	24.5 – 29.3	1.18
	About as active	50.1	1868	1.27	47.6 – 52.6	1.09
	Less active	23.0	1868	1.02	21.0 – 25.0	1.05
	When intends to take more exercise					
Men	Within the next month	23.1	1477	1.28	20.6 – 25.6	1.16
	Within the next six months	20.5	1477	1.06	18.4 – 22.6	1.01
	Within the next year	10.9	1477	0.83	9.3 – 12.5	1.02
	Intends to take more exercise but not in the next year	3.6	1477	0.48	2.7 – 4.5	0.98
	Unlikely to take more exercise	41.8	1477	1.48	38.9 – 44.7	1.15
Women	Within the next month	22.2	1865	1.28	19.7 – 24.7	1.33
	Within the next six months	23.9	1865	1.24	21.5 – 26.3	1.25
	Within the next year	10.5	1865	0.94	8.7 – 12.3	1.32
	Intends to take more exercise but not in the next year	2.9	1865	0.42	2.1 – 3.7	1.08
	Unlikely to take more exercise	40.4	1865	1.39	37.7 – 43.1	1.22
	Frequency of moderate-intensity activity for 30 minutes or more					
Men	Less than one day a week (sedentary)	25.8	1524	1.13	23.6 – 28.0	1.01
	1-2 days a week	23.8	1524	1.19	21.5 – 26.1	1.09
	3-4 days a week	11.3	1524	0.91	9.5 – 13.1	1.12
	5 or more days a week	39.0	1524	1.34	36.4 – 41.6	1.07
Men	Less than one day a week (sedentary)	26.4	1920	1.23	24.0 – 28.8	1.22
	1-2 days a week	29.0	1920	1.13	26.8 – 31.2	1.09
	3-4 days a week	14.6	1920	1.00	12.6 – 16.6	1.24
	5 or more days a week	30.1	1920	1.19	27.8 – 32.4	1.14

Table A.18 Standard errors and 95% confidence intervals for nutrition variables

Base	Characteristic	%(p)	Sample size	Standard error of p	95% confidence interval	Deft
	Whether thinks diet is different to a year ago					
Men	Diet is the same	82.2	1525	1.23	79.8 – 84.6	1.25
	Diet is difficult	17.5	1525	1.20	15.1 – 19.9	1.23
Women	Diet is the same	78.2	1920	1.14	76.0 – 80.4	1.21
	Diet is different	21.7	1920	1.14	19.5 – 23.9	1.21
	Whether eats meat or fish					
Men	Eats meat and fish	92.3	1525	0.85	90.6 – 94.0	1.25
	Eats meat only	5.1	1525	0.69	3.7 – 6.5	1.23
	Eats fish only	1.0	1525	0.23	0.5 – 1.4	0.91
	Eats neither meat or fish	1.6	1525	0.41	0.8 – 2.4	1.31
Women	Eats meat and fish	89.9	1920	0.85	88.2 – 91.6	1.24
	Eats meat only	4.3	1920	0.58	3.2 – 5.4	1.25
	Eats fish only	3.2	1920	0.48	2.3 – 4.1	1.19
	Eats neither meat or fish	2.6	1920	0.46	1.7 – 3.5	1.26
	Whether agrees that 'I get confused over what's supposed to be healthy and what isn't'					
Men	Agree	35.5	1523	1.40	32.8 – 38.2	1.14
	Disagree	49.5	1523	1.66	46.2 – 52.8	1.29
	Neither agree nor disagree	15.0	1523	1.08	12.9 – 17.1	1.18
Women	Agree	26.9	1920	1.10	24.7 – 29.1	1.09
	Disagree	60.5	1920	1.29	58.0 – 63.0	1.15
	Neither agree nor disagree	12.6	1920	0.87	10.9 – 14.3	1.14
	Whether agrees that 'eating healthy food is expensive'					
Men	Strongly agree	6.0	1523	0.75	45 – 7.5	1.23
	Agree	28.2	1523	1.48	25.3 – 31.1	1.28
	Neither agree nor disagree	19.1	1523	1.13	16.9 – 21.3	1.12
	Disagree	43.0	1523	1.47	40.1 – 45.9	1.16
	Strongly agree	3.7	1523	0.59	2.5 – 4.9	1.22
Women	Strongly agree	8.3	1918	0.71	6.9 – 9.7	1.13
	Agree	30.9	1918	1.26	28.4 – 33.4	1.19
	Neither agree nor disagree	12.9	1918	0.96	11.0 – 14.8	1.25
	Disagree	44.6	1918	1.28	42.1 – 47.1	1.12
	Strongly agree	3.4	1918	0.42	2.6 – 4.2	1.03

All Change? The Health Education Monitoring Survey one year on

Table A.19 Standard errors and 95% confidence intervals for sexual health variables

Base	Characteristic	%(p)	Sample size	Standard error of p	95% confidence interval	Deft
	Repondents' assessment of 'the risk of someone like me getting HIV (the AIDS) virus'					
Men	Very high	3.0	990	0.65	1.7 – 4.3	1.19
	Quite high	6.1	990	0.93	4.3 – 7.9	1.22
	Low	57.9	990	1.79	54.4 – 61.4	1.14
	There is no risk at all	27.9	990	1.64	24.7 – 31.1	1.15
	Don't know	5.0	990	0.74	3.6 – 6.5	1.07
Women	Very high	1.9	1230	0.41	1.1 – 2.7	1.06
	Quite high	4.2	1230	0.76	2.7 – 5.7	1.32
	Low	59.7	1230	1.41	56.9 – 62.5	1.01
	There is no risk at all	30.1	1230	1.29	27.6 – 32.6	0.98
	Don't know	4.1	1230	0.60	2.9 – 5.3	1.06
	Used a condom with a new partner					
Men		58.9	190	4.08	50.9 – 66.9	1.14
Women		52.6	181	4.30	44.2 – 61.0	1.15

Table A.20 Standard errors and 95% confidence intervals for behaviour in the sun variables

Base	Characteristic	%(p)	Sample size	Standard error of p	95% confidence interval	Deft
	How important it is to have a suntan					
Men	Very important	2.1	1334	0.46	1.2 – 3.0	1.17
	Fairly important	17.4	1334	1.16	15.1 – 19.7	1.12
	Not important	80.5	1334	1.26	78.0 – 83.0	1.16
Women	Very important	4.2	1746	0.55	3.1 – 5.3	1.14
	Fairly important	26.1	1746	1.31	23.5 – 28.7	1.25
	Not important	69.5	1746	1.36	66.8 – 72.2	1.23
	Whether sunburnt in last year and number of occasions					
Men	Once	16.8	1524	1.11	14.6 – 19.0	1.16
	Twice	6.0	1524	0.66	4.7 – 7.3	1.09
	Three times	1.8	1524	0.39	1.0 – 2.6	1.13
	Four or more	1.5	1524	0.42	0.7 – 2.3	1.35
	Not in last year	73.7	1524	1.24	71.3 – 76.1	1.10
	Can't remember	0.2	1524	0.11	0.0 – 0.4	1.05
Women	Once	14.5	1920	0.96	12.6 – 16.4	1.20
	Twice	3.6	1920	0.57	2.5 – 4.7	1.34
	Three times	1.0	1920	0.25	0.5 – 1.5	1.11
	Four or more	1.1	1920	0.27	0.6 – 1.6	1.14
	Not in last year	79.6	1920	1.12	77.4 – 81.8	1.22
	Can't remember	0.3	1920	0.14	0.0 – 0.6	1.10

Appendix B Cognitive question-testing for the Health Education Monitoring Survey (HEMS)

by Linda Mortimer, Qualitative Methods Unit, Social Survey Division, ONS

Background

As noted in Chapter 1, the first Health Education Monitoring Survey (HEMS) took place in 1995. Comparisons between the results of the first two years of the survey raised some interesting questions in relation to the data on self-reported stress and on physical activity. Levels of self-reported stress were higher in 1996 than in 1995, although most of the indicators measured by the survey did not change significantly between 1995 and 1996. It also appeared that this question might be measuring dimensions of health which were not being captured by the questions on self-reported general health and morbidity. Analysis of the data on physical activity raised concerns about whether respondents were using the terms 'physical activity' (which includes activity at work, walking, heavy housework or gardening) and 'exercise' interchangeably. The Health Education Authority therefore commissioned the Qualitative Methods Unit of SSD to carry out some cognitive question-testing on a number of questions on these two topics as an enhancement to the pilot study for the 1997 survey. The questions, together with the probes used in the qualitative interviewing, are included as an annex to this appendix.

Following the cognitive question testing SSD made a number of recommendations to the HEA for changing the questions. However, as the 1997 survey involved a follow-up interview, it was decided not to implement any of these recommendations for 1997. Analysis of data from the 1995 and 1996 surveys showed that even quite small changes in question wording could have a significant effect on estimates. It was important to know that any observed changes between 1996 and 1997 were real ones, and not an artefact of question wording.

Methodology

The cognitive interviewing approach to question testing was developed during the 1980's by survey methodologists and psychologists[1]. This approach pays explicit attention to the mental processes that respondents use to answer questions, as the main focus is on the questionnaire rather than on the entire survey process. In particular it can explore respondents' comprehension of a question, the strategies they use to retrieve relevant information from memory and the decision processes they follow when giving an answer. This information is elicited from respondents during a cognitive interview using prepared and spontaneous probes.

Interviewers trained in cognitive interviewing techniques first conducted the 1997 HEMS quantitative pilot interview with respondents. As in previous years, the pilot questionnaire included questions on self-reported stress, general health and morbidity; physical activity and exercise. These questions were unchanged from the 1996 HEMS. The interviewer then conducted the cognitive interview for the relevant parts of the questionnaire with respondents selected to ensure a mix of age and sex. Fourteen men and 16 women aged between 18 and 75, were chosen[2]. The whole interview, including the quantitative pilot, took an average of an hour and a half.

The cognitive part of the interview was tape-recorded, and later transcribed for analysis. In analysing the transcripts, the first stage was to identify recurrent and important themes that came from the data in relation to each question. The next stage was to create an index of these themes to use in labelling the data. The researcher then went through the transcripts marking when a theme appeared during the interview. These themes were summarised on a series of charts, allowing easy comparison across and within each respondent[3]. The age and sex of respondent were both considered during the analysis process. There appeared to be no difference for these two factors in the way different themes appeared during the interviews, and they have not been considered further in this report.

Cognitive question testing on self-reported stress

As noted earlier, although most of the indicators measured by the survey did not change significantly between 1995 and 1996, levels of self-reported stress were higher in 1996 than in 1995[4]. For the 1996 HEMS report, self-reported stress was analysed by self-reported general health and self-reported morbidity. Although respondents whose general health was not good, and those reporting a long-standing illness or disability were more likely than others to say they experienced a large or moderate amount of stress in the 12 months before interview, some of those with good general health and with no chronic condition also reported this level of stress. In addition, more than a third of men and almost half of women who reported good health or who said they had no long-standing illness or disability felt that the stress they had experienced had been harmful to their health.

As many commentators have pointed out[5], health is multi-dimensional; it can be 'good' in some respects and 'bad' in others.

It is possible that HEMS respondents were thinking of one dimension of health when asked about their 'health in general', another when saying whether they had a long-standing illness and yet another when asked about the effect of stress on their health. There was no way of knowing, from the 1996 HEMS data, whether the question on self-reported stress was measuring psychiatric morbidity which was not been picked up by the question on self-reported long-standing illness, or whether respondents felt that they could experience such levels of stress and still report good general health. The aim of the cognitive testing was to ask respondents to reflect on which aspects of their lives they were considering when answering the questions on stress.

B.3.1 Levels of self-reported stress

Ask all respondents
Looking at this card, which of these statements best describes the amount of stress or pressure you experienced in the past 12 months, that is since (today's date) 1996.

1	*Completely free of stress*
2	*Small amount of stress*
3	*Moderate amount of stress*
4	*Large amount of stress*
5	*Don't know*

This question required respondents to perform two tasks. Firstly, they needed to understand the terms 'stress' and 'pressure'; and they were therefore asked about their understanding of these terms. Secondly, they had to decide how much stress and pressure they had experienced over the last 12 months. The strategy they used to answer the question was explored.

'Pressure' was described by most respondents as being 'put on you' by others or by themselves. For many it came from having deadlines at work or from having more and more work to do. It was not seen by respondents as constant, but was thought to come and go as deadlines were met or problems solved. Pressure was thought to be positive by some respondents, as it 'gingers you up' and helped them to concentrate. Without pressure some felt they would not be able to work efficiently and quickly. However, pressure was seen as positive only while respondents felt they could 'manage it'.

'Stress' was seen by respondents as being caused by pressure. Stress itself was understood to be the feelings respondents experienced when under pressure. It was thought by respondents to come from inside and to affect people mentally and physically. When unable to cope with stress, respondents reported that they felt it was 'welling up inside', until they were 'keyed-up' and unable to continue with their 'normal course' of life. Interestingly, when discussing the terms stress and pressure, respondents used the term 'stress' interchangeably with pressure, even though they were able to define them clearly as two different terms.

Respondents were asked to explain what they understood by each answer category in this question. The first category, being 'completely free of stress', was thought by respondents to be something they only experienced when away from their normal life, perhaps on holiday, or lying on a beach. Someone who was completely free of stress was seen by respondents as having no problems at all. Respondents thought such a person would not to have 'a care in the world', or if they did have any problems, they would be able to cope without even seeing them as a problem. This was not seen as realistic by most respondents, and they asked whether such a person could exist.

A 'small amount of stress' was reported by respondents to be necessary to 'keep them going'. Some respondents thought a small amount of stress had a positive effect on them, as it helped to make them work harder. This level of stress was reported to come from everyday living or having just occasional problems. Respondents saw someone who experienced a small amount of stress as slightly stressed by everyday worries. Such a person was thought to be aware of problems but able to cope with them. The third answer category, 'a moderate amount of stress' was what some respondents felt they had all the time, and that it was sometimes containable and sometimes not. This level of stress was seen by most respondents as the point at which stress started taking over, where they reported feeling 'pressured'. Respondents felt they could not just 'get along' with a moderate amount of stress in their lives, and would have to make a decision to deal with stress at this level.

Respondents saw the 'large amount of stress' category as being when they were unable to cope, when things start 'getting on top of them'. A large amount of stress was thought by respondents to go on and on, until they were unable to perform their 'normal functions'. Some respondents talked about this being the point at which stress started to 'get bad'.

Respondents who experienced lower levels of stress saw people with larger amounts of stress in their lives as being exceptionally unsettled by stress and likely to find it difficult to cope. Respondents reported feeling that people with large amounts of stress would be affected both mentally and physically, causing them to be tense and stressed all the time. A few respondents who reported lower levels of stress felt that large amounts of stress could be self-induced; some people were seen as 'going looking for it', or 'putting themselves in the way of stress'.

B.3.2 The perceived effects of stress on health

Ask if the respondent reported stress in the last 12 months.
How harmful would you say the amount of stress and pressure you have experienced in the last 12 months has been to your physical and mental health? Has it been...

1	*very harmful*
2	*quite harmful*
3	*or not harmful at all?*
4	*Don't know*

Respondents showed a clear understanding of the way in which stress could be harmful. When asked what the term harmful meant in relation to stress, they talked in terms of stress causing physical problems such as high blood pressure, headaches, stomach pains and ulcers. The effects on mental health which were mentioned included disturbed sleep, irritability, agitation, easily becoming emotional and even suicidal.

When asked where they had found information about the harmful effects of stress, many respondents had read about stress and its effect in magazines and newspapers. Some had then discussed the issue with their friends and family. A small number had received information from their doctor.

Respondents were asked to explain what they understood by the answer categories used in this question. They saw the term 'very harmful' as the extreme end of stress-related symptoms. When stress had become very harmful it meant a breakdown; respondents thought that it would become difficult to hold down a job and they would need to get help, perhaps from a doctor. The physical effects of stress were interpreted as their bodies telling them they could not cope with the amount of stress they were experiencing. Respondents understood 'quite harmful' to be when stress does affect you, but you are still able to lead a normal life.

B.3.3 Other health questions

B.3.3.1 Health in general

Ask all respondents
Now I would like to ask you some questions about your health. How is your health in general? Would you say it was..

1	very good
2	good
3	fair
4	bad
5	or very bad?

When asked to define the term 'health in general' most respondents were able to say clearly what aspects of health they thought the term was referring to and mentioned a number of dimensions. 'Health in general' was seen as the absence of ill health. Respondents talked about not being sick, never getting colds, rarely needing to see a doctor or take time off work. 'Health in general' was also seen as related to the extent they felt their heath restricted their ability to live a normal life. To have good health in general meant to some respondents that their health did not prevent them from doing anything they wished to do. Respondents also referred to it as their state of mind, how they felt in themselves. 'Health in general' was also seen by respondents in terms of how 'fit' they thought they were, and was related to the amount of exercise taken and the type of diet followed.

Although the question does not reflect a specific time period, respondents were asked what time period they were considering when answering this question. Some respondents reported thinking about how their health had been over the last 12 months, either because some of the HEMS questions mention 'twelve months' or because they had just been asked to recall significant events over the previous 12 months[6]. Those who reported thinking of a different period of time considered their health over the last one to two months, while others reported thinking back across the last 'few' years and even their whole of their life. Some respondents even reported thinking of how their health was going to be in the coming months.

Although the question did not ask respondents to compare themselves with others, some did, usually comparing themselves to friends or family of a similar age but whose health was worse. Their response therefore included some relative assessment of health.

Respondents were asked to explain what they understood by each answer category in this question. Someone with 'very good' health in general was seen as having no restrictions on the things they could do. Such a person was thought by many respondents to have no health problems at all, and to be in exceptional condition for their age, again a relative assessment. Some respondents talked about such a person even being an Olympic athlete. Very good health in general was thought to be not only physical health but also mental health, both maintained by lots of exercise. Some saw no difference between 'very good' and 'good'.

The phrase 'good' health in general was understood by respondents to be referring to 'normal health', where they may have slight health problems such as colds or flu, or mental health problems that prevented them from being in very good health. Someone with good health was thought by respondents to be fit, but not an athlete.

The phrase 'fair' health in general was thought by respondents to be referring to health that was worse than good health, and that could be the average of good and bad 'health' days. Someone with fair general health would not be as fit as someone with good health, and might have a sedentary job. Respondents reported that there would be some restrictions to the things that someone with fair health could do, such a person would be more sickly and perhaps even need a short stay in hospital for some reason. However respondents thought that someone with 'fair health in general' could be worse.

The phrase 'bad' health in general was seen as applying to the negative aspects of health. Someone who had bad health was thought by respondents to have been ill for some time which would have made them unfit for work, again introducing a time dimension, and would restrict their ability to perform their 'daily tasks'. It was also seen as referring to smokers and drinkers, and people who do not know about fitness and diet. 'Very bad' health was thought to be severe and a condition that could affect all aspects of a person's life.

B.3.3.2 Long-standing Illness, disability and infirmity

Ask all respondents
Do you have any long-standing illness, disability or infirmity? By long-standing I mean anything that has troubled you over a period of time or that is likely to affect you over a period of time?

1	Yes
2	No

Respondents' understanding of the terms 'illness', 'disability' and 'infirmity' was explored during the cognitive interview. 'Illness' was seen by respondents as the extent to which normal life was restricted by minor illness, such as colds and coughs, or more serious ailments such as asthma. An illness was seen as either treatable, or something respondents thought they would recover from. Unlike the question on self-reported general health, this question did include a time dimension. The period of time that respondents thought someone needed to have had an illness for it to be long-standing varied greatly. Respondents did not express a strong opinion, mentioning periods ranging from a matter of months to the whole of someone's life. Some talked in terms of 'from the moment of diagnosis' or 'for rest of life'.

'Disability' was also thought of as a restriction on normal life, and respondents mentioned the term as referring to both mental and physical disabilities. They thought that someone could be born with a disability, or could acquire it through an accident. A disability was seen as permanent, and not thought by respondents to be curable.

Respondents had difficulty in explaining the term 'infirmity'. Whilst some associated it with old age, and used phrases such as the 'old and infirm', most either could not give a definition or saw it as interchangeable with illness and disability.

B.3.4 Discussion

It appears that respondents consider several factors or dimensions of health when answering questions on self-reported health and morbidity. Health in general appears to include absence of ill-health, the ability (or not) to lead a normal life, state of mind, and physical fitness. Any restrictions on normal life are seen as stemming from very *general* health problems, whereas long-standing illness is seen as the extent to which normal life is restricted by *specific* health problems.

Stress as a separate health dimension was not mentioned by respondents when discussing their health in general or with regard to a long-standing illness, disability or infirmity. It appears that stress was not considered by respondents as a factor in their health until the questions on stress mentioned the term.

Whether respondents felt they were leading a healthy life

B.4.1 Healthy life question

Ask all respondents
On the whole, would you say that you lead ...

1	*a very healthy life*
2	*a fairly healthy life*
3	*a not very healthy life*
4	*or an unhealthy life?*
5	*Don't know*

Data from all three HEMS surveys show that about 90% of men and women of all ages and social classes say they are leading a very healthy or fairly healthy life; this question therefore does not appear to discriminate between different groups of respondents. Respondents were asked what they understood by the term 'healthy life'. This was reported to be the extent to which active steps were being taken to achieve or maintain health or fitness. Respondents thought that how healthy they were was related to how healthy their diet was and how much exercise they took.

A minority of respondents reported leading a 'very healthy life'. When asked what they understood by this phrase, they explained that it meant they took regular exercise, tried to follow a healthy diet and tried to limit the amount they smoked or drank. Those who did not report leading a 'very healthy life' thought this category referred to those who were extreme or fanatical about their health; they did not break any of the 'rules'. The majority of respondents thought these 'rules' to be that they should always follow a very healthy diet, take plenty of exercise, and should not smoke or drink alcohol.

Most respondents felt they lived a 'fairly' healthy life, which they understood to be 'quite healthy'. They thought their life to be 'the middle of the road' and meant they took all things in moderation. They felt their lifestyle could be improved, but that it was not bad 'considering' their age, weight, the diet they followed, and whether they took any exercise.

Someone who lived a 'not very healthy life' was thought by the majority of respondents to be ailing and needing to do something about their health. Those who lived an 'unhealthy' life were seen by respondents as 'couch potatoes' and were thought actively to seek this kind of life.

Physical activity

The section on physical activity in the HEMS questionnaire contains several questions designed to measure respondents' perceptions of their own levels of activity and, in 1996, their knowledge of recommended levels of activity. Some questions use the term 'physical activity'; others refer to 'exercise'. About three quarters of HEMS respondents say they are very or fairly physically active 'compared with others of the same age', while about half feel they get enough exercise to keep fit. These proportions are at odds with the proportions who are actually active at the levels recommended for health gain, although previous qualitative work has shown that survey respondents assess themselves as 'fit enough' for a sedentary life[7,8]. About two thirds of HEMS respondents say they would like to take more exercise.

It is not possible to know from the data collected by HEMS whether respondents think 'exercise' and 'physical activity' have distinct meanings, or whether they are using the terms interchangeably. During the cognitive interview, respondents' understanding of these terms was explored.

B.5.1 Physical activity question

Ask all respondents
Compared to other people of your age would you describe yourself as..

1	*very physically active*
2	*fairly physically active*
3	*not very physically active*
4	*or not at all physically active?*

There appeared to be at least three interpretations of the term 'physically active'; actually being active, having the potential to be active, and being fit or not being restricted by being unfit. Some respondents described physical activity as being on the move, or keeping the body moving in some way or another. The types of activities all respondents referred to when describing the term 'physical activity' included running, walking, cycling, playing sports such as golf, football, squash, DIY, heavy housework, lifting and gardening.

When asked what they understood by the term 'very physically active' respondents reported seeing this as achieving a level of 'ultra, ultra fitness'. For most respondents this would involve personal 'exercise' on top of normal physical work and verged on the 'fanatical'. It was someone who 'climbs every mountain', who made a conscious effort to exercise at every opportunity. Respondents felt it would be difficult to keep up with a person like this. For respondents whose movements were restricted by injury, being very physically active would mean being able to do whatever they wanted without a care in the world.

The term 'fairly physically active' was seen by respondents as referring to being 'fairly' or 'pretty' fit. A person who was fairly fit was thought by respondents to have an active job, but not to exercise, or did exercise but worked in an office all day. Someone who was 'not very physically active' was thought not to play sports and to do lots of sitting around. Such a person was not thought to be interested in activity. They would get out of breath quickly when they did do something.

All Change? The Health Education Monitoring Survey one year on

95

Some saw the 'not at all physically active' as the same as 'not very'. Others talked about 'couch potatoes' who just sit in front of the television all the time. These people would be 'not active, not fit, need help' Respondents felt that such people made no effort to be physically active. A small number of respondents recognised that someone who was not at all physically active could have a disability, and therefore would not be able to do any activities.

B.5.2 Exercise question

Ask all respondents
On the whole, do you think you get enough exercise at present to keep you fit?

> 1   Yes
> 2   No
> 3   Can't take exercise

Respondents' understanding of the terms 'exercise' and 'fit' were examined, along with their view of what constitutes 'enough' exercise. For most respondents the term exercise referred to more than just, say, housework. They reported thinking that it involved increasing the heart rate and breaking out into a sweat[9], and that it was something they chose to do. The types of exercise these respondents described included swimming, running, and playing sports. For others, exercise came from doing housework or running up and down stairs all day at work.

For most, fitness was thought to be an individual thing that was dependent on their age and possibly their weight. It was seen by respondents as being what felt right for them, being able to do what they wanted to do and was related to their general well-being. For some this included not getting out of breath when being active, being able to jump up and do anything, and was related to being healthy.

How much exercise was thought to be 'enough exercise' was seen by respondents as being individual for each person. The majority of respondents talked about enough exercise being 'what's right for you', and there being 'no such concept' as a prescribed level of exercise that they should follow. A small number talked about elevating their heart rate for a period of time. Most felt it came down to what they felt comfortable with.

Data from the 1996 HEMS indicated that many respondents were aware of 'recommended levels of activity'; a quarter thought that people should be active for at least 30 minutes on five or more days a week, while over three fifths mentioned at least 20 minutes on three or more days a week. Nevertheless, the results of the cognitive interviewing suggest that not all respondents see the recommended levels relevant to them.

B.5.3 Exercise and physical activity

As all respondents had used the terms 'physically active' and 'exercise' interchangeably throughout the cognitive interview, they were asked to explain the difference between the two terms. Their explanations were confused and contradictory. The term 'exercise' was described by some as doing day-to-day tasks such as house-work, while for others it was doing things 'in addition' to house-work, such as going to the gym or taking part in sports. For some respondents 'physical activity' was understood to include cleaning and being active at work, and for others it was using their physical fitness attained through exercise to play sports. For a number of respondents there was no difference between physical activity and exercise, as both involved the use of the body's energy.

B.5.4 Wish to take more exercise

Ask all respondents
Would you like to take more exercise than you do at the moment?

> 1   Yes
> 2   No

During the main quantitative interview, respondents were asked about their intentions to take more exercise (see Appendix D and Chapter 5). The cognitive interview was concerned with how likely it was that respondents would **actually** increase the amount of exercise they do at the moment. Some felt that it was 'quite likely' they would do more exercise, but few could say that they would definitely be increasing the amount of exercise they did in the future. The likelihood of increasing their level of exercise was seen to depend on factors out of their control, such as recovering from illness or an injury. Others did not wish to increase their activity or felt it unlikely that they would as they already found it difficult to fit in what they did now.

B.5.5 Discussion

It appears respondents were aware of the HEA health promotion message to take exercise or physical activity, through magazines, newspapers and the television. However, it seems that the details of the message may not have got through, as respondents are not thinking of 'exercise' and 'physical activity' as distinct, but using the terms interchangeably.

Notes and references

1. Willis G B. Cognitive interviewing and questionnaire design: a training manual. Office of Research and Methodology, National Centre for Health Statistics, Working Paper series, No 7. March 1994.

2. In the context of the survey sample, the number of respondents participating in the cognitive question testing is small. However, the aim was not to select a large representative sample, but to explore the meanings and processes which respondents used when answering questions.

3. See Mortimer L. Qualitative research methods. *NHS Health Survey Advice Centre Survey Briefing* No 7. December 1996 pp 4-6 for a description of these methods.

4. Hansbro J et al. *Health in England 1996: what people know, what people think, what people do.* TSO (London 1997).

5. Blaxter M. *Health and Lifestyles.* Routledge (London 1990).

6. The questionnaire included a section asking about important life events in the 12 months between the two interview (see Appendix E). In the pilot, these questions were asked *before* the general health section of the interview, but were asked *afterwards* in the main fieldwork.

7. Killoran A et al; Who needs to know what? An investigation of the characteristics of the key target groups for the promotion of physical activity in England. In Killoran A et al (eds). *Moving on: international perspectives on promoting physical activity.* Health Education Authority (London 1994).

8. Wimbush E. A; Moderate approach to promoting physical activity: the evidence and implications. *Health Education Journal*, vol. 53, 1994, pp. 322-336.

9. This description may have been prompted by questions in the physical activity section of the interview which asked respondents whether the sports and exercise they engaged in had made them 'out of breath or sweaty'.

Annex B.1 HEMS questions and probe list

Mark the answer to each question as you conduct the HEMS pilot interview with the laptop. On completion, probe the respondents' understanding of the following questions. You may need to remind the respondent of the question and the answer they gave during the interview.

Genhlth   [*] Now I would like to ask you some questions about your health. How is your health in general? Would you say it was.
RUNNING PROMPT

     1   very good
     2   good
     3   fair
     4   bad
     5   or very bad?

Tell me in your own words what you understand by the term 'health in general'. What factors did you take into account when deciding how to answer this question-
     probe for   *- period of time considered*
            - whether compared self with others, who compared to and why.
            - specific events that influenced view of health,
            - are negative health events remembered more than positive events
What if any is the difference between
         - very good and good,
         - Bad and very bad
         - good and fair
         - Fair and bad

Illness   [*] Do you have any long-standing illness, disability or infirmity? By long-standing I mean anything that has troubled you over a period of time or that is likely to affect you over a period of time?

     1   Yes
     2   No

Tell me in your own words what you understand by the term(s) -
         - illness
         - disability
         - infirmity

How long do you need to have an illness, disability or infirmity for it to be long-standing?
What period of time did you consider when answering this question? How recent was this?
Were there any other periods of time you could have considered?
What factors did you take into account when deciding how to answer this question-
     probe for   *- whether compared self with others,*
            - who compared to and why.
            - whether included factors due to age

Hlthlife   [*] On the whole, would you say that you lead .
RUNNING PROMPT

     1   a very healthy life
     2   a fairly healthy life

     3   a not very healthy life
     4   or an unhealthy life?
     5   Don't know

How did you go about answering this question?
     probe for   *- period of time considered*
            - lifestyle, work habits
            - whether compared self with others,
            - who compared to and why.
            - did they compare themselves with how they were when younger
            - specific events that influenced view of health,

Are negative health events remembered more than positive events?
Do you take any active steps towards being healthy?
What, if any is the difference between
            very healthy and fairly healthy
            fairly healthy and not very healthy
            not very healthy and unhealthy life?

*If answer is **DON'T KNOW** - Why did you have difficulty answering this question?*

Stress   [*] Looking at this card, which of these statements best describes the amount of stress or pressure you experienced in the past 12 months, that is since (today's date) 1996.
SHOW CARD D

     1   Completely free of stress
     2   Small amount of stress
     3   Moderate amount of stress
     4   Large amount of stress
     5   Don't know

What, if any, is the difference between stress and pressure?
What factors did you consider when answering this question?
     Probe for   *- specific stressful events*
            - whether compared self with others,
            - who compared to and why.
            - Over what time period did they think about,

*If answer is **DON'T KNOW** - Why did you have difficulty answering this question? What, if any is the difference between*
            - being completely free of stress and having a small amount of stress
            - a small amount of stress and a moderate amount of stress
            - a moderate amount of stress and a large amount of stress?

Ask if Stress = 2-4

Harm   How harmful would you say the amount of stress and pressure you have experienced in the last 12 months has been to your physical and mental health? Has it been.
RUNNING PROMPT

     1   very harmful
     2   quite harmful
     3   or not harmful at all?
     4   Don't know

*How did you decide how to answer this question? How did you
decide what was due to pressure and what to stress?
Would you tell me in your own words what do you understand by
the term 'harmful'?
What factors did you consider when answering this question?*
> *Probe for   - physical effects
>   - mental effects*
*What, if any is the difference between
                  - very harmful and quite harmful
                  - quite harmful and not harmful at all
What information have they received about the effects of stress?
Where has this come from?*
> *Probe for   - TV, newspapers, magazines,
>   - Doctors, hospitals or other medical
>   source,
>   - any other source.*

Physical activity

CompAct   [*] Compared to other people of your age would
             you describe yourself as.
             RUNNING PROMPT

             1   very physically active
             2   fairly physically active
             3   not very physically active
             4   or not at all physically active?

*What do you understand by the term 'physically active'?
What did you think of when answering this question?*
> *Probe for   - who compared self to
>   - what is included as physical activity
>   - difference between very and fairly/ fairly
>   and not very/ not very and not at all
>   physically active
>   - where ideas of physical activity come
>   from (media / medicine etc.)*

EnufAct   [*] On the whole, do you think you get enough
             exercise at present to keep you fit?

             1   Yes
             2   No
             3   Can't take exercise

*Tell me in your own words what you understand by the term
'exercise'? What do you understand by the term 'fit'?
What do you think of as 'enough exercise'? What if any is the
difference between 'exercise' and 'physical activity'?*
> *Probe for   - period of time considered as 'at present'
>   - types of activity / exercise considered
>   - where ideas of fit / exercise come from
>   (media / medicine etc.)*

Ask if EnufAct = yes or no

LikeMore   [*] Would you like to take more exercise than you
             do at the moment?

             1   Yes
             2   No

What did you think of when answering this question?
> *Probe for   - obligation for taking exercise where
>   ideas of ideal amounts of exercise come
>   from (media / medicine etc.)*

Annexe B.2: Case Studies

Case Study 1 - The harmful effects of stress

Susan is in her mid 40's. She felt she had experienced a large
amount of stress in the last 12 months, brought about by increased
work deadlines. This she thought had caused her 'psychological
stress', and had been harmful to her health. The type of stress-
related health symptoms Susan reported experiencing included
high blood pressure and an inability to sleep, which she thought
had led to the severe headaches she had been having. Susan does
not believe the stress she has experienced has been very harmful,
only quite harmful.

> *'Quite harmful is when it obviously does have an effect,
> but you still manage to lead a reasonably normal life, but it still
> has some effect but you manage to carry on with these effects
> whether it is slight sort of trauma physically or psychologically.
> You manage to carry on really.'*

Case Study 2a - Understanding of Physical Activity and Exercise

June is in her early sixties. Twenty years ago she suffered a spinal
injury leaving her needing to use a walking stick to get around and
suffering almost constant pain, especially when sitting for long
periods.

June describes herself as 'fairly physically active'. She can walk
for short periods of time, and uses mobility buses and taxis to get
herself out and about. She likes to walk around the garden, to make
sure she has plenty of fresh air. Being fairly physically active to
June means that she has to think about whether she is up to going
out, whether she will need to take pain killers. June regards being
very physically active as being able to do what you want whenever
you want, which she was able to do before her accident.

Case Study 2b - Understanding of Physical Activity and Exercise

Michael is in his late 40's. He considers himself to be fairly
physically active as he swims regularly, goes to a local gym, does
heavy gardening and likes to take long walks.

Michael feels that fitness is related to age, and that people should
be realistic in the type and amount of exercise they try to do. To
Michael, the amount of exercise that constitutes 'enough' depends
on the individual; he does not believe there can be such a concept
for everyone.

> *'Enough exercise. Oh dear these questions. Well I think it
> has to be . . . what you feel is right for yourself as well. What's
> enough exercise? Well that's just to keep all your body moving I
> think. All your parts moving. And what's enough exercise? Well
> that's a lucid word isn't it. I can't answer that. I don't think there
> is such a word, such a concept as enough exercise because that's
> highly. I mean it depends on so much really. On how, what state
> you are in yourself. I mean if you are infirm one thing is enough
> isn't it really. I can't answer that.'*

Appendix C   Physical activity – Energy intensity categories and frequency measures for different types of activity

by Alison Walker

The indicators of participation in physical activity

Physical activity as measured by the Health Education Monitoring Survey included:

- 'home' activities, (housework, gardening and DIY)
- walking
- sports and exercise activities including cycling
- activity at work

Stair climbing and caring activities were not included.

Two HEA indicators of participation were used, based on the intensity and frequency of activity. Both indicators included an element of duration; activities in the sports and recreational category were included in the first summary only if they had lasted at least 30 minutes and in the second if they had lasted at least 20 minutes.

HEA suggested health promotion indicator: Percentage active at moderate or vigorous level for 30 minutes or more, five times a week

The first summary measure is based on occasions of 'moderate or vigorous' intensity activity, defined as having an energy cost of at least 5 kcals/min. This included:

- 'heavy' housework and 'heavy' gardening or DIY
- walks of 1-2 miles at a fast or brisk pace
- sports and exercise activities (including cycling) defined as having an energy cost of at least 5 kcals/min - see below
- occupational activity defined as involving at least moderate intensity activity - see below

A duration threshold of at least 30 minutes was applied to sports activities, and walking was included only if the walk was of 1-2 miles or more (described in the question as 'usually ... lasting for at least 30 minutes'). All other types of activity were included irrespective of duration.

HEA suggested health promotion indicator: Percentage of adults 16-74 active at a vigorous level for 20 minutes three times a week

The second summary measure of activity is based on occasions of 'vigorous' intensity activity, defined as having an energy cost of at least 7.5 kcals/min. By definition, sports and exercise activities and occupational activity were the only categories which could be classified as 'vigorous' activity - see below.

A duration threshold of at least 20 minutes was applied to sports activities.

Energy intensity categories and frequency measures by activity type

Home activities: Energy cost

Moderate 'Heavy' housework and 'heavy' gardening/DIY were both classified as moderate-intensity activities. Respondents were shown cards giving the following examples:

Walking with heavy shopping for more than 5 minutes, moving heavy furniture, spring cleaning, scrubbing floors with a scrubbing brush, cleaning windows, or other similar heavy housework.

Digging, clearing rough ground, building in stone/bricklaying, mowing large areas with a hand mower, felling trees, chopping wood, mixing/laying concrete, moving heavy loads, refitting a kitchen or bathroom or any similar heavy manual work.

Home activities: Frequency

Number of days in the past four weeks on which informant did 'heavy' housework plus number of days on which did 'heavy' gardening/DIY.

Occupational activity: Energy cost

Vigorous Considers self 'very physically' active in job and is in one of the following occupations defined as involving heavy work, including:

fishermen/women, furnace operators, rollermen, smiths, forgers, faceworking coal-miners, construction workers, fire service officers, metal plate workers, shipwrights, riveters, steel erectors, benders, fitters, galvanisers, tin platers, dip platers, plasterers, roofers, glaziers, general building workers, road surfacers, stevedores, dockers, goods porters, refuse collectors.

Moderate Considers self 'very physically' active in job and is **not** in occupation groups listed above
OR
considers self 'fairly physically' active in job and is in one of the occupations listed above.

Occupational activity: Frequency

Not collected for occupational activity.

Sports and exercise activities: Energy cost

Vigorous
a) All occasions of running/jogging, squash, boxing, kick boxing, skipping, trampolining

b) Sports coded as vigorous intensity if they had made the respondent breathe heavily or sweat a lot, but otherwise coded as moderate intensity including: cycling, aerobics, keep fit, gymnastics, dance for fitness, weight training, football, rugby, swimming, tennis, badminton.

Moderate
(a) See 'vigorous' category (b), but where the activity did not make the respondent breathe heavily or sweat a lot.

(b) All occasions of a large number of sports including: basketball, canoeing, fencing, field athletics, hockey, ice skating, lacrosse, netball, roller skating, rowing, skiing, volleyball

c) Sports coded as moderate intensity if they had made respondent breathe heavily or sweat a lot, but otherwise coded as light intensity, including: exercises (press-ups, sit-ups etc), dancing.

Sports and exercise activities: Frequency and duration

Number of days in past four weeks.
Time usually spent per day of activity.

Walking: Energy cost

Moderate Walks of 1-2 miles or more with a brisk or fast pace.

Walking: Frequency

Number of walks of 1-2 miles or more in the past four weeks.

Reference period

A four-week reference period was used in the interview. Frequency of activity during the four-week period is expressed in the results as an average frequency per week, based on the following conversion:

Frequency of activity in past four weeks	Average frequency per week
0-3 days	Less than one day a week
4-11 days	1-2 days a week
12-19 days	3-4 days a week
20+ days	5 or more days a week

Modifications to the physical activity questions between 1995 and 1996

Some modifications were made to the questions on reported participation between the 1995 HEMS and the 1996 HEMS. These are described in detail in the 1996 report[1]. It is possible that one effect of these changes was to increase the reported frequency of participation in walking and thereby increase the overall frequency of participation in physical activity. This may account for the apparent increase seen in the trend tables between 1995 and 1996.

Measuring change

Section 5.3.1 describes the rationale behind the methods used to describe change. Two main summaries of change were used: change in the frequency of participation in different types of activity and change from one grouped frequency band to another. Both types of summary excluded change of less than one day per week (i.e. less than 4 days in the past four weeks).

Change in frequency

frequency in specified activity increased:
frequency in 1997 > frequency in 1996 by at least 4 days in past four weeks
frequency in specified activity decreased:
frequency in 1997 < frequency in 1996 by at least 4 days in past four weeks
frequency in specified activity changed by less than one day a week:
the difference between frequency in 1997 and frequency in 1996 is less than 4 days in the past four weeks.

Change in activity group

Activity group increased by at least one day a week:
the difference between frequency in 1997 and frequency in 1996 is at least 4 days in the past four weeks and:

frequency in 1996	frequency in 1997
less than one day a week	1-2 days a week or 3-4 days a week or 5+ days a week
1-2 days a week	3-4 days a week or 5+ days a week
3-4 days a week	5+ days a week

Activity group decreased by at least one day a week:
the difference between frequency in 1997 and frequency in 1996 is at least 4 days in the past four weeks and:

frequency in 1996	frequency in 1997
1-2 days a week	less than one day a week
3-4 days a week	less than one day a week or 1-2 days a week
5+ days a week	less than one day a week or 1-2 days a week or 3-4 days a week

Changed by less than one day a week:
the difference between frequency in 1997 and frequency in 1996 is less than 4 days in the past four weeks.

References

1. Hansbro J et al. *Health in England 1996: what people know, what people think, what people do.* Appendix C . TSO (London 1997).

Appendix D   Technical appendix

Logistic regression

Logistic regression is a multivariate statistical technique which has been used in a number of chapters in this report. It predicts the outcome of a dependent variable which only has two possible outcomes, for example being a current smoker and not being a current smoker, from a set of independent variables. Variables with only two possible outcomes are also known as dichotomous variables or binary variables Logistic regression was developed specifically for dichotomous variables and makes more appropriate assumptions about the underlying distributions and the range of possible proportions than the more familiar multiple linear regression method.

Most of the tables in the HEMS report (for example Table 2.1) are based on crosstabulations. These tables show the proportion of people with a given characteristic who display the behaviour of interest; an example would be the proportion of people aged 16-24 who smoke. What such tables do not show, however, is how much other factors may interrelate with the independent variable; for example, how much social class and sex may interrelate with age to influence whether or not a person smokes. Logistic regression looks at how different independent variables interrelate by looking at the odds of the behaviour occurring for different combinations of the independent variables. Odds refers to the ratio of the probability that the event will occur to the probability that the event will not occur. The odds can be converted into a probability (p) using the following formula:

$$p = \frac{\text{odds}}{1 + \text{odds}}$$

Logistic regression can therefore be used to predict the probability of a behaviour occurring given a combination of characteristics, for example, it can be used to model the probability of a person being either a smoker or a non-smoker given their age, sex and social class.

The logistic regression model can be written as

$$Prob(event) = \frac{e^z}{1 + e^z}$$

where e is the base of the natural logarithms. Logistic regression actually models independent variables against the log odds (the natural logarithm of the odds) of an event because this forms a linear relationship.

$$Z = B_0 + B_1X_1 + \ldots\ldots B_pX_p.$$

where the Xs are the independent variables, Bs are the model parameters and B_0 is the baseline odds. The odds of engaging in behaviour can then be calculated by multiplying the baseline odds by the appropriate factors.

Before carrying out the logistic regression analysis data are crosstabulated to give an indication of which independent variables should be included in the regression. One of the categories of each of the independent variables is then defined as a reference category (with a value of 1); the reference category is the group least likely to display the behaviour of interest. For each of the independent variables included in the regression a coefficient is produced which represents the factor by which the odds of a person taking part in the behaviour increases if the person has that characteristic. The odds produced by the regression are relative odds, that is they are relative to the reference category. Taking the example above, where smoking is the dependent variable, the age group 65-74 would be defined as the reference category as this is the group least likely to smoke and the odds given by the model would be relative to this; so it would be possible to say how much greater the odds were of a person aged 16-24 being a smoker than the odds of a person aged 65-74 being a smoker.

There are different methods of including independent variables in the logistic regression model. The method used in the HEMS analysis was forward stepwise selection which is where the model starts off only containing the constant and then at each step the independent variable which is the most highly significant is added in. Variables are then examined and the coefficients which make the observed results 'most likely' are selected while the others are removed using either the Wald statistic or the Likelihood-Ratio test. The Likelihood-Ratio test was used in the HEMS analysis.

The odds ratios produced by the regression are presented in the report as 'multiplying factors' and they are shown with the 95% confidence intervals. If the confidence interval does not include 1.00 then the odds ratio is likely to be significantly different from the reference category.

For a more detailed description of logistic regression analysis see Chapter 2 of *SPSS Advanced Statistics User's Guide* (SPSS Inc. 1990).

HEALTH EDUCATION MONITORING FOLLOW-UP SURVEY 1997

HOUSEHOLD BOX

Ask all respondents

IntTyp96   INTERVIEWER: THIS WAS A (Full.proxy) INTERVIEW
            LAST YEAR PRESS 1 TO CONTINUE

IntType   Code whether interview is full or proxy

            1   Full
            2   Proxy

IntType2   CODE WHETHER THIS IS A FACE-TO-FACE OR
            TELEPHONE INTERVIEW

            1   Face-to-face interview
            2   Telephone interview

W2Move   INTERVIEWER CODE: Has the informant (Name)
            moved to a new address since the last interview?.

            1   Yes
            2   No

If no feed forward data

NPerAd   I would like to start by asking you about yourself and
            your household. How many people normally live in this
            household?
            INCLUDE ALL PERSONS, INCLUDING THOSE AGED
            75 AND OVER:

            1..20

Ask/check for everyone in the household

Name   START WITH SELECTED PERSON
            ASK THE FOLLOWING QUESTIONS OF EVERY
            ONE IN THE HOUSEHOLD.

            Name or other identifier

Sex   INTERVIEWER: CODE NAME's SEX.

            1   Male
            2   Female

W2Status   INTERVIEWER CODE OR ASK: Please code the
            status of (name of person):

            1   Selected person
            2   is still a member of selected person's present
                household
            3   has moved out of selected persons household
            4   selected person has moved and (Name) still lives at
            5   has died
            6   is a new household member
            7   person is mistakenly listed

Ask check for selected person

DOB   INTERVIEWER: CODE SELECTED PERSONS'S
            DATE OF BIRTH.

            (DATE)

If aged 16 or over

Marstat   Are you/ is NAME ...

            1   married
            2   living as married
            3   single/never married
            4   widowed
            5   divorced
            6   or separated?
            7   SPONTANEOUS living with a same sex partner

Ask if informant is single, widowed, divorced or separated and aged 55 or under

Partner   May I just check, do you have a regular partner who
            does not live in the household?

            1   Yes
            2   No

Ask about everyone in the household

ReltoInf   ASK OR CODE RELATIONSHIP TO SELECTED
            PERSON

            1   Informant
            2   Spouse\partner (incl. same-sex partner)
            3   Son\daughter (incl. adopted/step-child)

4   Foster child
5   Son-in-law\daughter-in-law
6   Parent\step-parent
7   Parent-in-law
8   Brother\sister (incl. adopted)
9   Brother-in-law\sister-in-law
10   Grandchild
11   Grandparent
12   Other (related)
13   Other (not related)

If aged 16 or over

WhoHOH   IS THIS PERSON THE HOH?
REMEMBER THAT WHERE A PROPERTY IS
OWNED\RENTED IN THE NAME OF A WOMAN
WHO IS MARRIED\COHABITING WITH A MAN, THEN
BY DEFINITION, THE MAN IS THE HOH.

1   Yes
2   No

Ask all respondents

NewPers   INTERVIEWER: ASK OR CODE
Apart from that, is there anyone else - including any
children or babies - currently living in your household?

1   Yes
2   No

(If yes above a new line is opened in the household box to enter the details
of the next person)

Ask all respondents

NpersW2   THERE IS/ARE (number) PERSON\PEOPLE IN THE
HOUSEHOLD AT WAVE 2. IS THIS CORRECT? IF
YES PRESS ENTER TO CONTINUE, ELSE GO BACK
TO THE HOUSEHOLD BOX AND ADD OTHER
HOUSEHOLD MEMBERS

1..20

Ask if informant has been livinhg with partner for less than one year

Livtgth2   Can I just check, in which month did you start living
together as a couple?
ENTER MONTH

Ask all respondents

WorkLast   Did you do any paid work in the week ending last
Sunday, either as an employee or as self-employed?

1   Yes
2   No

If working last week

Fullpart   In your present job do you work

1   full-time
2   or part-time?

Ask if has moved sinced wave1

WhenMove   (You have moved address since we last interviewed
you,)
May I just check, when did you move?

(Date)

Ask all respondents

Ownorent   Does your household own or rent this accommodation?
CODE FIRST THAT APPLIES ..

1   Buying with a mortgage
2   Owned outright
3   Rented from Local Authority/New Town
4   Rented from Housing Association
5   Rented unfurnished
6   Rented furnished
7   Rented from employer
8   Other with payment

Ask if has moved in past year or new informant

AccomTyp   INTERVIEWER CODE TYPE OF ACCOMMODATION

1   Detached house
2   Semi-detached house
3   Terraced/end of terraced house
4   Purpose built flat
5   Flat in a converted house
6   Caravan, mobile home or houseboat
7   Other type of accomodation

Car   Is there a car or van **normally** available for use by you
or any members of your household?

1   Yes
2   No

GENERAL HEALTH

Ask all respondents

Genhlthw2   [*] Now I would like to ask you some questions about
your health. How is your health in general? Would you
say it was..
RUNNING PROMPT

1   very good
2   good
3   fair
4   bad
5   or very bad?

Illnesw2   [*] Do you have any long-standing illness, disability or
infirmity? By long-standing I mean anything that has
troubled you over a period of time or that is likely to
affect you over a period of time?

1   Yes
2   No

Lmatter   [*] What is the matter with you?

Limitact   [*] Does this illness or disability (Do any of these illnesses or disabilities) limit your activities in any way?

    1   Yes
    2   No

Ask all respondents

Goodhlw2   [*] Here is a list of factors that could affect your health. Which, if any, currently have a good effect on your health?
                  SHOW CARD A

    1   Relationships, family
    2   My work
    3   My income/standard of living
    4   My alcohol consumption
    5   The exercise I do
    6   What I eat
    7   None of these

Badhlw2   [*] Now I would like you to look at this card. Which of these, if any, currently have a bad effect on your health?
                  SHOW CARD B

    1   Not having a job
    2   Relationships, family
    3   Pollution
    4   My smoking
    5   Others' smoking
    6   My alcohol consumption
    7   Lack of exercise
    8   What I eat
    9   My weight
    10 None of these

Ask of women aged 16-49

Pregnant   May I just check, are you pregnant at the moment?

    1   Yes
    2   No
    3   DK

Ask of married or cohabiting men and same-sex cohabiting women, with a partner aged 16-49

Pregnt2   May I just check, is your wife/partner pregnant at the moment?

    1   Yes
    2   No
    3   DK

Ask all respondents

Hlthlfw2   [*] On the whole, would you say that you lead ...
                  RUNNING PROMPT

    1   a very healthy life
    2   a fairly healthy life

    3   a not very healthy life
    4   or an unhealthy life?
    5   Don't know

HlthIntr   Here are are some things people have said about health. I'd like you to say how far you agree with each statement, choosing your answer from this card.
                  SHOW CARD C

                  PRESS ENTER TO CONTINUE

Hlthimp   SHOW CARD C
life.   [*] To have good health is the most important thing in

    1   Strongly agree
    2   Agree
    3   Neither agree nor disagree
    4   Disagree
    5   Strongly disagree

Docsay   SHOW CARD C
                  [*] It's sensible to do exactly what the doctors say.

    1   Strongly agree
    2   Agree
    3   Neither agree nor disagree
    4   Disagree
    5   Strongly disagree

Hlthluck   SHOW CARD C
                  [*] Generally health is a matter of luck.

    1   Strongly agree
    2   Agree
    3   Neither agree nor disagree
    4   Disagree
    5   Strongly disagree

Toomuch   SHOW CARD C
                  [*] If you think too much about your health you are more likely to be ill.

    1   Strongly agree
    2   Agree
    3   Neither agree nor disagree
    4   Disagree
    5   Strongly disagree

Illdoc   SHOW CARD C
                  [*] I have to be very ill before I go to the doctor.

    1   Strongly agree
    2   Agree
    3   Neither agree nor disagree
    4   Disagree
    5   Strongly disagree

Dontthnk   SHOW CARD C
                  [*] I don't really have time to think about my health.

    1   Strongly agree
    2   Agree
    3   Neither agree nor disagree
    4   Disagree
    5   Strongly disagree

Stressw2 [*] Looking at this card, which of these statements best describes the amount of stress or pressure you experienced in the past 12 months, that is since (today's date) 1996.
SHOW CARD D

1 Completely free of stress
2 Small amount of stress
3 Moderate amount of stress
4 Large amount of stress
5 Don't know

Ask if Stressw2 = 2-4

Harmw2 How harmful would you say the amount of stress and pressure you have experienced in the last 12 months has been to your physical and mental health? Has it been...
RUNNNING PROMPT

1 very harmful
2 quite harmful
3 or not harmful at all?
4 Don't know

EVENTS CALENDAR

Ask all respondents

EventInt Now I would like to ask you about some of the things you have done since we last interviewed you.
On the whole would you say the last year has been...
RUNNING PROMPT:
1 good
2 average
3 or bad?
4 SPONTANEOUS: can't say

Wevent1 SHOW CARD E
Now I would like you to look at this card and say which of these things if any have happened to you in the past 12 months.
CODE ALL THAT APPLY

1 Got married/started new relationship
2 Had a baby
3 Had a serious operation illness or injury
4 Close friend/relative had serious illness or injury
5 Death of close relative or friend
6 Separation or breakup of a relationship
7 Problems with neighbours
8 Retired started new job changed jobs
9 Lost your job/ partner lost job
10 Problems at work
11 Serious financial problems
12 Personal experience of theft mugging or other crime
13 Family problems
14 Other event
15 None of these

If married/started a new relationship in the past 12 months

Whmar When did (you get married start new relationship)?
ENTER CODE(s) FOR MONTH
CODE ALL THAT APPLY

5 May 1996
6 June 1996
7 July 1996
8 August 1996

9 September 1996
10 October 1996
11 November 1996
12 December 1996
13 January 1997
14 February 1997
15 March 1997
16 April 1997
17 May 1997
18 June 1997
19 July 1997
20 All year
21 DOES NOT APPLY

If had a baby in the past 12 months

WhBab When did you have a baby?
ENTER CODE(S) FOR MONTH
CODE ALL THAT APPLY
(codes as above)

If had serious operation, illness or injury in past 12 months

WhIll When did you have a (serious operation illness or injury)?
ENTER CODE(S) FOR MONTH
CODE ALL THAT APPLY
(codes as above)

If close friend/relative had serious operation, illness or injury in past 12 months

WhIllOth When did your close relative/friend have a serious illness or injury?
ENTER CODE(S) FOR MONTH
CODE ALL THAT APPLY
(codes as above)

If close friend/relative has died

WhDeath When did your close relative or friend die?
ENTER CODE(S) FOR MONTH
CODE ALL THAT APPLY
(codes as above)

If separated /relationship broke up

WhSep When (did you separate/was the break-up of your relationship)?
ENTER CODE(S) FOR MONTH
CODE ALL THAT APPLY
(codes as above)

If had problems with neighbours

WhNeigh When did you have problems with neighbours?
ENTER CODE(S) FOR MONTH
CODE ALL THAT APPLY
(codes as above)

If retired/started new job/changed jobs

WhJob When did you (retire start a new job/change jobs)?
ENTER CODE(S) FOR MONTH
CODE ALL THAT APPLY
(codes as above)

If informant/partner lost job

Whlost   When did you (or your partner) lose your/their job?
ENTER CODE(S) FOR MONTH
CODE ALL THAT APPLY
(codes as above)

If had problems at work

WhWork   When did you have problems at work?
ENTER CODE(S) FOR MONTH
CODE ALL THAT APPLY
(codes as above)

If had serious financial problems

WhFin   When did you have serious financial problems?
ENTER CODE(S) FOR MONTH
CODE ALL THAT APPLY
(codes as above)

If experienced theft, mugging or other crime

WhTheft   When did you experience a theft, mugging or other crime?
ENTER CODE(S) FOR MONTH
CODE ALL THAT APPLY
(codes as above)

If has had problems with family

WhFam   When were the problems with your family?
ENTER CODE(S) FOR MONTH
CODE ALL THAT APPLY
(codes as above)

If has had other event

WhOther   When did ....(other event) happen?
ENTER CODE(S) FOR MONTH
CODE ALL THAT APPLY
(codes as above)

SMOKING

Ask all respondents

Smokintr   The following questions are about smoking.

PRESS ENTER TO CONTINUE

SmokeSC   INTERVIEWER: 16 AND 17 YEAR OLDS **MUST** SELF-COMPLETE
FOR INFORMANTS AGED 18 OR OVER THE QUESTIONS SHOULD BE ASKED BY YOU UNLESS YOU THINK THE INFORMANTS WOULD PREFER TO ANSWER THESE QUESTIONS BY SELF-COMPLETION

1   Completed by interviewer
2   Self-completion accepted and completed

Ask if SmokeSC = Accepted

SmkIntr2   I would like you to take the computer and answer the questions yourself. Instructions on how to answer the questions are given on the screen.

WORK THROUGH THE FIRST QUESTION WITH THE INFORMANT. IF THE INFORMANT MAKES A MISTAKE, TAKE THEM BACK TO THE QUESTION AND ALLOW THEM TO KEY IN THE RIGHT ANSWER.

Practice   Do you enjoy using computers?

1   Yes
2   No
3   Don't want to answer

If Cigevw1 (fed-forward) = No

W2Cigev   Have you ever smoked a cigarette, a cigar or a pipe?

1   Yes
2   No

Ask if Cigevw1 = yes (fed-forward) or W2CigEv = Yes

Cignoww2   Do you smoke cigarettes at all nowadays?

1   Yes
2   No

Ask if Cignoww2 = yes

Qtywkend   About how many cigarettes **a day** do you usually smoke at weekends?
IF LESS THAN 1, ENTER 0.

Qtywkday   About how many cigarettes **a day** do you usually smoke on weekdays?
IF LESS THAN 1, ENTER 0.

Cigtype   Do you mainly smoke...
RUNNING PROMPT

1   filter-tipped cigarettes,
2   plain or untipped cigarettes,
3   or hand-rolled cigarettes?

Ask if Cigtype = Handrolled

QtyTob   How much tobacco do you usually smoke **per week**?
Would you prefer to give your answer in

1   quarter ounces
2   or in grammes?

Ask if Qtytob = Ounces

QtyTobI   ENTER NO. OF **QUARTER** OUNCES PER WEEK
IF ANSWER GIVEN IN OUNCES, MULTIPLY BY FOUR
IF LESS THAN QUARTER OF AN OUNCE, ENTER 0.

0..20

Ask if Qtytob = Grams

QtyTobM   ENTER NO. OF GRAMMES PER WEEK

0..150

Nosmokw2	[*] How easy or difficult would you find it to go without smoking for a whole day. Would you find it... RUNNING PROMPT

1   very easy
2   fairly easy
3   fairly difficult
4   or very difficult?
5   Don't know

Ask if Cignoww2 = no

CigYear	Have you smoked a cigarette in the last year, that is since (today's date 1996)?

1   Yes
2   No

If CigYear = Yes

CigReg	[*] Did you smoke cigarettes.. RUNNING PROMPT

1   regularly, that is at least one cigarette a day
2   or did you smoke them only occasionally?
3   **SPONTANEOUS** Never really smoked cigarettes, just tried them once or twice.

Ask if CigReg = Regular

CigUsed	About how many cigarettes did you smoke in a **day** when you smoked them regularly? IF LESS THAN 1, ENTER 0.

IF CigNoww2 = Yes

Trystw2	In the last 12 months, that is since (today's date 1996) have you tried to give up smoking?

1   Yes
2   No

Ask if Trystw2 = yes OR Cigreg = regularly

NumStSmk	(You have now given up smoking. Including this time,) how many times have you tried to give up in the last year? USE CALENDAR TO PROMPT INFORMANT'S MEMORY

1..97

Ask about the last two occasions if Trystw2 = yes

StSmkInt	Now I would like to ask you about the last time/time before that when you tried to give up smoking.
WhenStSm	When did you try to give up? ENTER DATE
WhenSt	And when did you start smoking again? ENTER DATE
Lasttime	May I just check, how long was it for?

1   Less than a day
2   A day, less than a week
3   A week, less than a month
4   A month, less than two months

5   Two months less than three months
6   Three months than six months
7   Six months less than a year
8   One year or more

WhyStSmk	What was the **main** reason for giving up smoking then? DO NOT PROMPT

1   Own specific health problem
2   Own health generally
3   Health of children/other family members
4   Cost
5   Partner gave up
6   Pregnant/partner pregnant
7   Advised to by health professional
8   Other

Ask if WhyStSmk = Other

XwhyStSm	Please specify other reasons for giving up.
StSmkAid	Here is a list of things that people use to give up smoking. Which, if any, did you use? SHOW CARD F CODE ALL THAT APPLY

1   Nicotine chewing gum
2   Nicotine patch
3   Special clinic or stop smoking group
4   Quitline
5   Will power
6   Advice from a doctor, or other health professional
7   Support from family and friends
8   Other
9   None of these

Ask about the last two occasions if CigReg = Regular

StSmkInt	Now I would like to ask you about when you gave up smoking this time/ the time before that when you tried to give up smoking.
WnStSm2	When did you (try to) give up? ENTER DATE

Ask for previous attempt to give up smoking only

WhenSt2	And when did you start smoking again? ENTER DATE
Lasttim2	May I just check, how long was it for?

1   Less than a day
2   A day, less than a week
3   A week, less than a month
4   A month, less than two months
5   Two months less than three months
6   Three months less than six months
7   Six months less than a year
8   One year or more

Ask about the last two occasions if CigReg = Regular

WhyStSm2	What was the **main** reason for giving up smoking then? DO NOT PROMPT (Codes as for whystsmk)

XwyStSm2   Please specify other reasons for giving up.

StSmAid2   Here is a list of things that people use to give up
            smoking. Which, if any, did you usen then?
            SHOW CARD F
            CODE ALL THAT APPLY

            1   Nicotine chewing gum
            2   Nicotine patch
            3   Special clinic or stop smoking group
            4   Quitline
            5   Will power
            6   Advice from a doctor, or other health professional
            7   Support from family and friends
            8   Other
            9   None of these

Ask if Cignoww2 = yes

TryCut   And in the last year, that is since (today's date 1996)
            have you tried to cut down on your smoking?

            1   Yes
            2   No

If Try cut = yes

Cutstp   [*] When you last tried to cut down on smoking, were
            you....
            RUNNING PROMPT

            1   Cutting down as a first step towards stopping or
                were you
            2   just cutting down?

CigLess   [*] On the whole, do you think you are smoking
            RUNNING PROMPT

            1   more
            2   about the same
            3   or fewer cigarettes than you did a year ago?
            4   Didn't smoke a year ago

If Cigless = more or didn't smoke a year ago

Wymorles   Is there any particular reason why you are smoking
            more than a year ago?/
            What is the main reason you started smoking regularly
            in the last year?

            1   To lose weight
            2   Stress
            3   Pressure from friends/colleagues
            4   Lack of will power
            5   Enjoy it
            6   Boredom
            7   Other
            8   No particular reason

If Cignoww2 = yes

Giveupw2   [*] Would you like to give up smoking altogether?

            1   Yes
            2   No
            3   Don't know

Ask if Giveupw2 = yes

Stop1   Now I would like you to look at this card, and say which
            of the statements best describes you.
            SHOW CARD G

            1   I intend to give up smoking within the next month
            2   I intend to give up smoking within the next six
                months
            3   I intend to give up smoking within the next year
            4   I intend to give up smoking, but not in the next year
            5   I'm unlikely to give up smoking

Ask if Giveupw2 = no or don't know

Stop2   Now I would like you to look at this card, and say which
            of the statements best describes you.
            SHOW CARD H

            1   I'm unlikely to give up smoking
            2   I intend to give up smoking within the next month
            3   I intend to give up smoking within the next six
                months
            4   I intend to give up smoking within the next year
            5   I intend to give up smoking, but not in the next year

If has ever smoked at wave 1 but does not smoke now and has not smoked in the past year

IntCigAg   You told us last year that you have smoked in the past,
            can I just check
            PRESS ENTER TO CONTINUE

If Cigevw1 = Yes or W2CigEv = Yes

CigAge   How old were you when you started to smoke
            cigarettes regularly?
            ENTER 0 IF NEVER SMOKED CIGARETTES
            REGULARLY

            0..97

If CigNoww2 = NO and CigYear = 2 (ie. gave up more than a year ago)

AgeGave   And how old were you when you last gave up smoking?
            ENTER 0 IF NEVER SMOKED CIGARETTES
            REGULARLY

            0..97

Ask if (CigNoww2= yes)

Homesmw2   Do you ever smoke at home?

            1   Yes
            2   No

Ask if married, or living with someone

Partsmk2   Does your husband/wife/partner smoke ?

            1   Yes
            2   No
            3   Don't know

Ask if informant doesn't smoke at home and partner smokes or more than two people in household or doesn't have partner in houshold

Anysmkw2   Does anyone in the household (including your partner) smoke at home at all nowadays?

1   Yes
2   No

DRINKING

Ask all respondents

DrnkIntr   I'd now like to ask you some questions about what you drink - that is, if you do drink.
PRESS ENTER TO CONTINUE

DrinkNow   Do you ever drink alcohol nowadays, including drinks you brew at home?

1   Yes
2   No

Ask if Drinknow = no

DrinkAny   Could I just check, does that mean you never have an alcoholic drink nowadays, or do you have an alcoholic drink very occasionally, perhaps for medicinal purposes or on special occasions like Christmas or New Year?

1   Very occasionally
2   Never

Ask if Drinkany = never

TeeTotal   Have you always been a non-drinker, or did you stop drinking for some reason?

1   Always a non-drinker
2   Used to drink but stopped

If TeeTotal = 2

StopDrk   May I just check, did you stop drinking
RUNNING PROMPT

1   during the last year
2   or was it more than a year ago?
3   SPONTANEOUS Cant remember

If StopDrk = in the last year

WhenStDrk   When did you stop drinking?
ENTER CODE FOR MONTH

WhyStdrk   What was the **main** reason for giving up drinking?
DO NOT PROMPT

1   Own specific health problem
2   Own health generally
3   Cost
4   Pressure from family
5   Was affecting my/others life
6   Pregnant

7   Advised to by health professional
8   Change in work situation/social life
9   Other

Ask if Drinknow = yes or DrinkAny = very occasionally

Drtyintr   I'd like to ask you whether you have drunk different types of alcoholic drink in the last 12 months. I do not need to know about non-alcoholic or low alcohol drinks.

PRESS ENTER TO CONTINUE

Shandy   SHOW CARD I
How often have you had a drink of ...... SHANDY (exclude bottles/cans) during the last 12 months, that is since (today's date) 1996

1   Almost every day
2   5 or 6 days a week
3   3 or 4 days a week
4   once or twice a week
5   once or twice a month
6   once every couple of months
7   once or twice a year
8   not at all in the last 12 months

Ask if has drunk shandy

ShandyAm   How much .... SHANDY (exclude bottles/cans) have you usually drunk on any one day during the last 12 months, that is since (today's date) 1996?
ENTER NUMBER OF **HALF** PINTS.

Ask if Drinknow = yes OR Drinkany = very occasionally

Beer   SHOW CARD I
How often have you had a drink of ...BEER, LAGER, STOUT, CIDER during the last 12 months, that is since (today's date) 1996?

1   Almost every day
2   5 or 6 days a week
3   3 or 4 days a week
4   once or twice a week
5   once or twice a month
6   once every couple of months
7   once or twice a year
8   not at all in last 12 months

Ask if has drunk beer

BeerAm   Other than cans or bottles, How many HALF PINTS of BEER, LAGER, STOUT, CIDER, have you usually drunk on any one day during the last 12 months, that is since (today's date) 1996?
ENTER NUMBER OF **HALF** PINTS.
IF YOU NORMALLY DRINK CANS OR BOTTLES, ENTER 97

Ask if Beeram = 97

XBeeram   (Please write in) how many bottles or cans (do) you normally drink on one day. For example, 3 large cans or 2 small cans. (Ask the interviewer for help if you are not sure.)

Spirits   SHOW CARD I
How often have you had a drink of ... SPIRITS OR
LIQUEURS (eg. gin, whisky, rum, brandy, vodka,
advocaat) during the last 12 months, that is since
(today's date) 1996?

1   Almost every day
2   5 or 6 days a week
3   3 or 4 days a week
4   once or twice a week
5   once or twice a month
6   once every couple of months
7   once or twice a year
8   not at all in last 12 months

Ask if has drunk spirits

SpiritAm   How much .... SPIRITS OR LIQUEURS (eg. gin,
whisky, rum, brandy, vodka, advocaat) have you
usually drunk on any one day during the last 12
months, that is since (today's date) 1996?
ENTER NUMBER OF SINGLES (COUNT DOUBLES
AS TWO SINGLES).

Ask if Drinknow = yes OR Drinkany = very occasionally

Sherry   SHOW CARD I
How often have you had a drink of ... SHERRY OR
MARTINI (including port, vermouth, cinzano, dubonnet)
during the last 12 months, that is since (today's date)
1996?

1   Almost every day
2   5 or 6 days a week
3   3 or 4 days a week
4   once or twice a week
5   once or twice a month
6   once every couple of months
7   once or twice a year
8   not at all in last 12 months

Ask if has drunk sherry

SherryAm   How much .... SHERRY OR MARTINI (including port,
vermouth, cinzano, dubonnet) have you usually drunk
on any one day during the last 12 months, that is since
(today's date) 1996?
ENTER NUMBER OF SMALL GLASSES

Ask if Drinknow = yes OR DrinkAny = Very occasionally

Wine   SHOW CARD I
How often have you had a drink of ... WINE (including
babycham, champagne) during the last 12 months,
that is since (today's date) 1996?

1   Almost every day
2   5 or 6 days a week
3   3 or 4 days a week
4   once or twice a week
5   once or twice a month
6   once every couple of months
7   once or twice a year
8   not at all in last 12 months

Ask if has drunk wine

WineAm   How much .... WINE (including babycham, champagne)
have you usually drunk on any one day during the last
12 months, that is since (today's date) 1996?
ENTER NUMBER OF GLASSES

Ask if Drinknow = yes OR DrinkAny = Very occasionally

Lemon   SHOW CARD I
How often have you had a drink of ... ALCOHOLIC
LEMONADE, ALCOHOLIC COLA OR OTHER
ALCOHOLIC SOFT DRINKS during the last 12 months,
that is since (today's date) 1996?

1   Almost every day
2   5 or 6 days a week
3   3 or 4 days a week
4   once or twice a week
5   once or twice a month
6   once every couple of months
7   once or twice a year
8   not at all in last 12 months

Ask if has drunk alcoholic lemonade/cola or other alcoholic soft drinks

XLemonAm   How much .... ALCOHOLIC LEMONADE, ALCOHOLIC
COLA OR OTHER ALCOHOLIC SOFT DRINKS have
you usually drunk on any one day during the last 12
months, that is since (today's date) 1996?
ENTER AMOUNT...

Ask if Drinknow = yes OR DrinkAny = Very occasionally

Ifother   SHOW CARD I
Have you had any other alcoholic drinks during the last
12 months, that is since (today's date) 1996?

1   Yes
2   No

Ask if Ifother = yes

XIfother   Please say which other kind of drink you have had.

Otherd   SHOW CARD I
How often have you had a drink of ...OTHER during the
last 12 months, that is since (today's date) 1996?

1   Almost every day
2   5 or 6 days a week
3   3 or 4 days a week
4   once or twice a week
5   once or twice a month
6   once every couple of months
7   once or twice a year
8   not at all in last 12 months

OtherAm   How much of ....OTHER have you usually drunk on any
one day during the last 12 months, that is since (today's
date) 1996?
ENTER AMOUNT...

Droftw2   SHOW CARD I
           Now I would like you to think about alcoholic drinks of
           all kinds. How often would you say you had an alcoholic
           drink of any kind?

           1   Almost every day
           2   5 or 6 days a week
           3   3 or 4 days a week
           4   once or twice a week
           5   once or twice a month
           6   once every couple of months
           7   once or twice a year
           8   not at all in last 12 months

If drinks once or twice a week or more

TriedCut   Have you tried to cut down on or stop drinking in the
           last 12 months, that is since (date 12 months ago)?

           1   Yes
           2   No

If TriedCut = Yes

NumCtDrk   How many times have you tried to cut down on or stop
           drinking in the last year?
           USE CALENDAR TO PROMPT INFORMANT'S
           MEMORY

           1..97

Ask about the last two occasions tried to cut down on drinking

CtDrkInt   Now I would like to ask you about the last time/time
           before that when you tried to cut down on or stop
           drinking.

WhenCtDr   When did you try to cut down/stop?
           ENTER CODE FOR MONTH

HowCtDrk   [*] Did you stop drinking altogether, drink on fewer days
           each week, or drink less when you did drink?
           CODE ALL THAT APPLY

           1   Stop drinking altogether
           2   drink on fewer occasions each week
           3   or drink less when you did drink?

WhyCtdrk   What was the **main** reason for trying to cut down?
           DO NOT PROMPT

           1   Own specific health problem
           2   Own health generally
           3   Cost
           4   Pressure from family
           5   Was affecting my/others life
           6   Pregnant
           7   Advised to by health professional
           8   Change in work situation/social life
           9   Other

All who drink at all

DrAmount   [*] On the whole, would you say that you are drinking ..
           RUNNING PROMPT

           1   more
           2   about the same
           3   or less than you did a year ago?

If drinking less than a year ago and have not tried cutting down

Whyless   What is the **main** reason you are drinking less than a
           year ago?
           DO NOT PROMPT

           1   Own specific health problem
           2   Own health generally
           3   Cost
           4   Pressure from family
           5   Was affecting my/others life
           6   Pregnant
           7   Advised to by health professional
           8   Change in work situation/social life
           9   Other

If Dramount = more

WhydMor   [*] Is there any particular reason why you are drinking
           more than a year ago?

           1   Stress,
           2   Mixing with people who drink more,
           3   Better off financially,
           4   Its good for you/health reasons,
           5   Enjoy it,
           6   No particular reason,
           7   Other

Ask if 1-4 at DrOftw2

LikeCw2   [*] On the whole would you say that you drink
           RUNNING PROMPT

           1   about the right amount
           2   or would you like to drink less?

If LikeCw2 Less

dStop1   Now I would like you to look at this card, and say which
           of the statements best describes you.
           SHOW CARD J

           1   I intend to cut down my drinking within the next
                month
           1   I intend to cut down my drinking within the next six
                months
           2   I intend to cut down my drinking within the next year
           3   I intend to cut down my drinking, not in the next year
           4   I'm unlikely to cut down on my drinking

PHYSICAL ACTIVITY

Ask all respondents

ExerIntr   I'd like to ask you about some of the things you have
           done (at work or) in your free time that involve physical
           activity in the past 4 weeks.
           SHOW THE LAST FOUR WEEKS ON THE CALENDAR

           PRESS ENTER TO CONTINUE

If not working last week

Wrklast4   Can I just check, have you done any paid work in the
           last 4 weeks either as an employee or as self-employed?

           1   Yes
           2   No

Active   Thinking about your job in general, (ASK ABOUT MAIN JOB ONLY) would you say that you are ....
RUNNING PROMPT

1   very physically active
2   fairly physically active
3   not very physically active
4   or not at all physically active in your job?

Ask all respondents

HouseWrk   (I'd like you to think about physical activities you have done when you were not doing your paid job.)
Have you done any housework in the past 4 weeks?

1   Yes
2   No

Ask if Housewrk = yes

HWrkList   SHOW CARD K
Have you done any housework listed on this card?

1   Yes
2   No

Ask if Hwrklist = yes

HevyHWrk   SHOW CARD L
Some kinds of housework are heavier than others. This card gives examples of heavy housework, it does not include everything, these are just examples. Was any of the housework you did in the past 4 weeks this kind of heavy housework?

1   Yes
2   No

Ask if HevyWrk = yes

HeavyDay   During the past 4 weeks on how many separate days have you done that kind of heavy housework?

Ask all respondents

Garden   (Apart from at work) Have you done any gardening, DIY or building in the past 4 weeks?

1   Yes
2   No

Ask if Garden = yes

GardList   SHOW CARD M
Have you done any gardening, DIY or building work listed on this card?

1   Yes
2   No

Ask if Gardlist = Yes

ManWork   SHOW CARD N
Have you done any gardening, DIY or building work from this card, or any similar heavy manual work?

1   Yes
2   No

Ask if Manwork = yes

ManDays   During the past 4 weeks, on how many days have you done this kind of heavy manual gardening or DIY?

Ask all respondents

WalkPre   I'd like you to think now about all the walking you've done in the past 4 weeks, either locally or away from here. Include any country walks, walking to and from work, and any other walks that you have done.

PRESS ENTER TO CONTINUE

WalkB   Have you done any walks of a quarter of a mile or more in the past 4 weeks? That would usually be continuous walking lasting 5 to 10 minutes.

1   Yes
2   No
3   Can't walk at all

Ask if WalkB = yes

MileWlkB   Did you do any walks of 1-2 miles or more in the past 4 weeks? That would usually be continuous walking for at least 30 minutes.

1   Yes
2   No

Ask if MileWlkB = yes

MileNumB   During the past 4 weeks how many times did you do any walks of 1-2 miles or more?

1..97

WalkPace   Which of the following best describes your usual walking pace..
RUNNING PROMPT

1   a slow pace
2   a steady average pace
3   a fairly brisk pace
4   or a fast pace - at least 4 mph?

Ask all respondents

ActAny   SHOW CARD O
Now I'd like you to think about any sports or exercise activities you do. Can you look at this card and tell me if you've done any of these types of activities during the past 4 weeks?

1   Yes
2   No

Ask if Actany = yes

WhchAct   Which of the activities did you do?
CODE ALL THAT APPLY
SHOW CARD O

1   Aerobics/keep fit/gymnastics
2   Bowls/Crown bowls
3   Circuit training/weight training

4 Cycling
5 Dancing
6 Exercises
7 Football
8 Golf
9 Hiking
10 Hockey/Netball/Ice-skating
11 Jogging/Running/Athletics
12 Squash
13 Swimming
14 Tennis/Badminton
15 Any other sport or exercise activity like these
16 Any other sport or exercise activity like these

If WhchAct = Other (15 or 16)

XWhchAc1/   SPECIFY OTHER ACTIVITY
XWhchAc2   (You can specify two extra types)

Ask about any activities which the informant has done

Occ   Can you tell me on how many separate days did you (name of activity) during the past 4 weeks?

TimeAct   How much time did you usually spend (name of activity) on each day?
ENTER TIME IN MINUTES
IF MORE THAN ONE HOUR, CALCULATE TIME IN MINUTES

Effort   During the past four weeks, was the effort of (name of activity) enough to make you feel out of breath **or** sweaty?

1 Yes
2 No

EnufAcw2   [*] On the whole, do you think you get enough exercise at present to keep you fit?

1 Yes
2 No
3 Can't take exercise

Ask if EnufAct = yes or no

ActYear   [*] On the whole, would you say that you are
RUNNING PROMPT

1 more active
2 about as active
3 or less active than you were a year ago?

LikeMow2   [*] Would you like to take more exercise than you do at the moment?

1 Yes
2 No

Ask if Likemow2 = Yes

Exermor1   Now I would like you to look at this card, and say which of the statements best describes you.
SHOW CARD P

1 I intend to take more exercise within the next month
2 I intend to take more exercise within the next six months
3 I intend to take more exercise within the next year
4 I intend to take more exercise, but not in the next year
5 I'm unlikely to take more exercise

Ask if Likemow2 = no or don't know

Exermor2   Now I would like you to look at this card, and say which of the statements best describes you.
SHOW CARD Q

1 I'm unlikely to take more exercise
2 I intend to take more exercise within the next month
3 I intend to take more exercise within the next six months
4 I intend to take more exercise within the next year
5 I intend to take more exercise, but not in the next year

Ask all respondents

Stpexw2   SHOW CARD R
Here is a list of things that people say stops them getting more exercise. Looking at this card, could you please tell which, if any, apply to you.
CODE ALL THAT APPLY

1 I don't have the time
2 I have an injury or disability that stops me.
3 My health is not good enough.
4 I don't enjoy physical activity.
5 I'm not the sporty type.
6 Other
7 None of these

NUTRITION

Ask all respondents
Dietintr   Now I would like to ask you a few questions about the sorts of food you eat and drink.
PRESS ENTER TO CONTINUE.

DietChn   [*] On the whole, would you say that the sorts of things that you eat and drink are
RUNNING PROMPT

1 the same as
2 or different from a year ago?
3 Don't know

If 'different' at DietChn

HowChn   [*] In what way have the things that you eat and drink changed in the last year?
DO NOT PROMPT
CODE ALL THAT APPLY

1 Eat fewer sweets, cakes, puddings, chocolate,
2 Eat less fatty food/fried foods, snacks,
3 Eat more fruit and vegetables,
4 Stopped eating meat,
5 Eat more pasta, rice, bread, beans,
6 Eat more fatty foods, snacks, fast foods,
7 Eat a special diet e.g. because of diabetes, allergies, anaemia,
8 Cut down on alcohol,
9 Other

XOthSpec   Please specify other ways in which the sorts of things that you eat and drink have changed in the past year:

WhyChD [*] What is the main reason that the sorts of things that you eat and drink have changed in the last year?
DO NOT PROMPT:

1 Concerns about food safety
2 To lose weight/maintain weight
3 Specific health reason
4 Other health reason
5 Cost
6 Ethical reasons
7 Other

Ask all respondents

VegInt Now I would like to ask you whether you ever eat certain types of food.
PRESS 1 TO CONTINUE

EatMeat ASK OR CODE   Can I just check, do you ever eat meat nowadays?
INCLUDE ALL RED AND WHITE MEAT AND PROCESSED MEATS SUCH AS SAUSAGES, BURGERS AND MEAT PIES DO NOT INCLUDE FISH

1 Yes
2 No

EatFish And do you ever eat fish?
INCLUDE SHELLFISH

1 Yes
2 No

Eatdairy And do you ever eat dairy foods including eggs?
INCLUDE PREPARED FOODS WITH DAIRY INGREDIENTS:

1 Yes
2 No

Ask all respondents

ChgeHbw2 SHOW CARD S
[*] Which one of these statements best describes how you feel about the sorts of food you eat nowadays?

1 I have never felt any need to change what I eat
2 I have already changed as much as I am going to
3 I feel that I ought to make changes but probably won't
4 I am likely to make changes in the future.

Ask all respondents

Agrehlth Now I am going to read you a list of statements. I would like you to say whether you agree or disagree with them, choosing your answer from this card
SHOW CARD T

PRESS ENTER TO CONTINUE

HlthFood SHOW CARD T
[*] Eating healthy food is expensive.

1 Strongly agree
2 Agree
3 Neither agree nor disagree
4 Disagree
5 Strongly disagree

Tasty SHOW CARD T
[*] The tastiest foods are the ones that are bad for you.

1 Strongly agree
2 Agree
3 Neither agree nor disagree
4 Disagree
5 Strongly disagree

EnjyHlth SHOW CARD T
[*] Healthy foods are enjoyable.

1 Strongly agree
2 Agree
3 Neither agree nor disagree
4 Disagree
5 Strongly disagree

WhatHlth SHOW CARD T
[*] I get confused over what's supposed to be healthy and what isn't.

1 Strongly agree
2 Agree
3 Neither agree nor disagree
4 Disagree
5 Strongly disagree

ExpertOp SHOW CARD T
[*] Experts never agree about what foods are good for you.

1 Strongly agree
2 Agree
3 Neither agree nor disagree
4 Disagree
5 Strongly disagree

Dietw2 [*] Thinking overall about the things you eat, would you say that your diet is..
RUNNING PROMPT..

1 as healthy as it could be
2 quite good but it could improve
3 or not very healthy?
4 Don't know

Ask if 2-4 at diet

HlthDw2 [*] Would you like to eat a healthier diet than you do at the moment?

1 Yes
2 No
3 Don't know

If yes at hlthdw2

ChDietw2 Now I would like to look at this card and say which of the statements best describes you:
SHOW CARD U

1 I intend to change my diet within the next month
2 I intend to change my diet within the next six months
3 I intend to change my diet within the next year
4 I'm unlikely to change my diet

SKIN CANCER

Ask all respondents

IntroSc   There's been a lot of publicity recently about skin cancer. I would like to ask you a few questions about this.
PRESS ENTER TO CONTINUE

Creamsw2   Do you ever wear a suncream?

1   Yes
2   No
3   Never go out in the sun

Ask if Creamsun = Yes

Whencrem   When do you use a suncream?
Please choose your answers from this card.
SHOW CARD V
CODE ALL THAT APPLY

1   Sunbathing abroad
2   Outdoors abroad, but not sunbathing
3   Sunbathing in this country
4   Outdoors in this country doing something else

Ask all respondents

SunBurw2   During the last 12 months, that is since (today's date) 1996, have you had sunburn causing redness and soreness of the skin lasting for at least 1-2 days?

1   Yes
2   No
3   Can't remember

Ask if Sunburn = yes

FreqBurn   How many times?

1   Once
2   Twice
3   Three times
4   Four or more
5   Not in the last 12 months

Ask if has white or olive skin (answer 1 or 4 at Skntypw1, fed-forward)

SunTanw2   [*] How important is having a suntan to you personally? Is it..
RUNNING PROMPT

1   very important
2   fairly important
3   or not important?
4   Don't know

CLASSIFICATION

The qualifications and ocupation and industry questions in this section are fed-forward and checked with informants.

Ask all respondents

Demintr   Now I would like to ask you a few more questions about yourself.

PRESS ENTER TO CONTINUE

Quals1   May I just check, have you ever passed any exams?

1   Yes
2   No

Ask if Quals1 = yes

Quals2   SHOW CARD W

Please look at this card and tell me the first exam you come to that you have passed.

1   Degree or equivalent
2   Teaching or other higher qualification
3   A level or equivalent
4   GCSE, O level or equivalent
5   CSE or equivalent
6   CSE ungraded
7   Other qualifications

Origin   SHOW CARD X
[*] To which of the groups on this card do you consider you belong?
1   White
2   Black Caribbean
3   Black African
4   Black Other
5   Indian
6   Pakistani
7   Bangladeshi
8   Chinese
9   None of these

Ask if aged under 55

Student   May I just check, since Easter this year, apart from leisure classes, have you studied full-time at a school or college, or university ?

1   Studied full-time at school/college
2   Studied full-time at university
3   Has not studied full-time at school/college or university

Ask if not in paid work in the last week and if female and aged under 63 or male and aged under 65

Scheme   You said earlier that you were not in paid work last week, can I just check, were you on a government scheme for employment training?

1   Yes
2   No

All Change?   The Health Education Monitoring Survey one year on

115

JBAway   (You said earlier that you were not in paid work last week)
Did you have a job or business you were away from?

1   Yes,
2   No
3   **SPONTANEOUS** Waiting to take up a new job/ business already obtained

Ask if JBAway = No or waiting to take up job

UnPaid   Did you do any unpaid work in that week for any business that you own?

1   Yes
2   No

Ask if Unpaid = No

Rel   .....or that a relative owns?

1   Yes
2   No

Ask if Rel = No

Start4   Thinking of the four weeks ending last Sunday were you looking for any kind of paid work or government training scheme at any time in those four weeks?

1   Yes
2   No

Ask if Start4 = yes

LKTima   How long have you been looking for paid work/ a place on a government scheme?

1   less than one month
2   1 month but less than 3 months
3   3 months but less than 6 months
4   6 months but less than 12 months
5   12 months but less than 18 months
6   18 months but less than 2 years
7   2 years but less than 3 years
8   3 years but less than 4 years
9   4 years but less than 5 years
10 5 years or more

Ask if Start4 = Yes

Start2   If a job or a place on a government scheme had been available in the week ending last Sunday would you have been able to start work within two weeks?

1   Yes
2   No

Ask if Start4 = No or Start2 = No

NoLook   What was the main reason you did not seek any work in the last four weeks/would not be able to start in the next two weeks?

1   Student
2   Looking after the family/home
3   Temporarily sick or injured
4   Long-term sick or disabled
5   Retired from paid work
6   Other reasons

Ask if not working last week, but not retired or missing/don't know at scheme - start2

Everpaid   (Apart from the job you are waiting to take up) Have you ever been in paid employment?

1   Yes
2   No

Ask if working last week, has ever worked or retired

IndD   What does/did the firm/organisation you work/ed for mainly make or, do (at the place where you worked)?
DESCRIBE FULLY - PROBE MANUFACTURING or PROCESSING or DISTRIBUTION ETC. AND MAIN GOODS PRODUCED, MATERIALS USED, WHOLE SALE or RETAIL ETC

IndT   ENTER A TITLE FOR THE INDUSTRY

OccT   What is/was your (main) job (in the week ending last Sunday?)
ENTER JOB TITLE

OccD   What did/do you mainly do in your job?
CHECK SPECIAL QUALIFICATIONS/TRAINING NEEDED TO DO THE JOB

RecJob   CODE WHETHER YOU HAVE JUST HAD TO MAKE ANY CHANGE AT ALL TO INDUSTRY (IndD or IndT) OR OCCUPATION (OccD or OccT).

1   Neither industry nor occupation changed at all
3   Both changed
5   Only industry changed
7   Only occupation changed
8   COMPUTED: New Socinfo

Stat   Are/were you working as an employee or are/were you self-employed?

1   Employed
2   Self-employed

Ask if Stat = employed

Manage   ASK OR RECORD
Did/do you have any managerial duties, or are/were you supervising any other employees?

1   Manager
2   Foreman/supervisor
3   Not manager/supervisor

EmpNo   How many employees are/were there at the place where you work/ed?

1   1-24
2   25 or over+

Ask if stat = self-employed

Solo   ASK OR RECORD
Are/were you working on your own or did/do you have
employees?

    1   On own/with partner(s) but no employees
    2   With employees

Ask if Solo = with employees

SENo   How many people did/do you employ at the place
where you work/ed?

    1   1-24
    2   25 or over

Ask if informant is not HOH

HOHIntro   I would now like to talk about HOH's employment.

          PRESS ENTER TO CONTINUE

HWorklst   May I just check, did HOH do any paid work in the week
ending last Sunday, either as an employee or as self-
employed?

    1   Yes
    2   No

Ask if HOH not in paid work in the last week and if female and aged under 63 or male and aged under 65

HScheme   Was HOH on a government scheme for employment
training?

    1. Yes
    2. No

Ask if HScheme = No OR female and aged 63 or over or male and aged 65 or over (and not in paid work)

HJBAway   Did HOH have a job or business he/she was away from?

    1   Yes,
    2   No
    3   **SPONTANEOUS** Waiting to take up a new job/
business already obtained

Ask if HJBAway = No

HUnPaid   Did HOH do any unpaid work in that week for any
business that he/she owns?

    1   Yes
    2   No

Ask if HUnpaid = No or waiting to take up a job

Hrel   .....or that a relative owns?

    1   Yes
    2   No

Ask if Hrel = No

Hstart4   Thinking of the four weeks ending last Sunday was
HOH looking for any kind of paid work or government
training scheme at any time in those four weeks?

    1   Yes
    2   No

Ask if Hstart4 = yes

HStart2   If a job or a place on a government scheme had been
available in the week ending last Sunday would HOH
have been able to start work within two weeks?

    1   Yes
    2   No

Ask if Hstart4 = No OR Hstart2 = No

HNoLook   What was the main reason HOH did not seek any work
in the last four weeks/would not be able to start in the
next two weeks?

    1   Student
    2   Looking after the family/home
    3   Temporarily sick or injured
    4   Long-term sick or disabled
    5   Retired from paid work
    6   Other reasons

Ask if HOH was not working last week, but not retired or missing/don't know at Hscheme - Hstart2

HEverpd   (Apart from the job he/she is waiting to take up) Has
HOH ever been in paid employment?

    1   Yes
    2   No

Ask if HOH was working last week or has ever had a job

HIndD   What does/did the firm/organisation HOH worked for
mainly make or do (at the place where HOH worked)?
DESCRIBE FULLY - PROBE MANUFACTURING or
PROCESSING or DISTRIBUTION ETC. AND MAIN
GOODS PRODUCED, MATERIALS USED, WHOLE
SALE or RETAIL ETC

HIndT   ENTER A TITLE FOR THE INDUSTRY

HOcct   What was HOH's (main) job (in the week ending last
Sunday?
ENTER JOB TITLE

HOccD   What does HOH mainly do in his/her job?
CHECK SPECIAL QUALIFICATIONS/TRAINING
NEEDED TO DO THE JOB

HRecJob   CODE WHETHER YOU HAVE JUST HAD TO MAKE
ANY CHANGE AT ALL TO INDUSTRY (IndD or IndT)
OR OCCUPATION (OccD or OccT).

    1   Neither industry nor occupation changed at all
    3   Both changed
    5   Only industry changed
    7   Only occupation changed
    8   COMPUTED: New Socinfo

HStat	Was HOH working as an employee or was he/she self-employed?	5	£15,000 - £19,999 £300-£399
		6	£20,000 - £29,999 £400-£599
	1 Employee	7	£30,000 or more £600 or more
	2 Self-employed	8	Don't know

HStat   Was HOH working as an employee or was he/she
self-employed?

1   Employee
2   Self-employed

Ask if HStat = employed

HManage   ASK OR RECORD
Did HOH have any managerial duties, or was he/she
supervising any other employees?

1   Manager
2   Foreman/supervisor
3   Not manager/supervisor

HEmpNo   How many employees are/were there at the place
where HOH works/ed?

1   1-24
2   25 or over

Ask if HStat = self-employed

HSolo   ASK OR RECORD
Is/was HOH working on his/her own or does/did he/she
have employees?

1   On own/with partner(s) but no employees
2   With employees

Ask if Hsolo = with employees

HSENo   How many people does/did HOH employ at the place
where he/she works/ed?

1   1-24
2   25 or over

INCOME

Ask all respondents

Benefits   Are you or anyone else in your household receiving any
of the following state benefits?
CODE ALL THAT APPLY

1   Income support
2   Family credit
3   Housing benefit
4   None of these
5   Don't know

TotHhInc   SHOW CARD Y
The next question is on income. Choose the number
from this card which represents the group in which you
would place your TOTAL HOUSEHOLD INCOME from
all sources BEFORE tax and other deductions.
(EXPLAIN IF NECESSARY: INCOME FOR LAST
TWELVE MONTHS)

Per Year   Per Week
1   Under £2,500   Under £50
2   £2,500 - £4,999   £50-£99
3   £5,000 - £9,999   £100-£199
4   £10,000 - £14,999   £200-£299

5   £15,000 - £19,999   £300-£399
6   £20,000 - £29,999   £400-£599
7   £30,000 or more   £600 or more
8   Don't know
9   SPONTANEOUS: Nothing
10   SPONTANEOUS: Refused

DRUG USE

Ask those aged 16-55 if face-to-face interview

Nonresp   The following sections is self-completion. I would like
you to take the computer and answer the questions
yourself. Instructions on how to answer the questions
are given on the screen.
WORK THROUGH THE FIRST QUESTION WITH
THE INFORMANT
IF THE INFORMANT MAKES A MISTAKE, TAKE
THEM BACK TO THE QUESTION AND ALLOW THEM
TO KEY IN THE RIGHT ANSWER.

HAS THE INFORMANT THE ACCEPTED
SELF-COMPLETION?

1. Self-completion accepted and completed
2. Completed by interviewer
3. All self-completion refused (drugs and sexual health)
4. Informant refused drugs self-completion but
    completed sexual health
5. Informant refused sexual health self-completion
    but completed drugs

Ask if Nonresp = refused all self-completion or refused drugs or refused sexual health

Whyrefd   INTERVIEWER - CODE REASON WHY INFORMANT
REFUSED

1   Didn't like computer
2   Eyesight problems
3   Other disability
4   Objected to subject
5   Worried about confidentiality
6   Could not read or write
7   Ran out of time
8   Language problems
9   Couldn't be bothered
10   Other - Specify at next question

Ask if Whyrefd = 10

XWhyrefd   Specify reasons for refusal.

Ask if Nonresp = self-completed or accepted and completed by interviewer

Practice   Do you enjoy using a computer

1   Yes
2   No
3   Don't want to answer

Intro2   The following questions are about drugs. Please
          answer them honestly. THE ANSWERS YOU GIVE
          ARE COMPLETELY CONFIDENTIAL. The questions
          ask whether or not you have ever used drugs. If you are
          not sure what you have taken, there are a couple of
          questions at the end that cover this. Please do not
          include drugs prescribed by a doctor.
          To go to the next question now, PRESS 1 for YES and
          PRESS THE RED BUTTON

DRQ1A   Have you EVER taken AMPHETAMINES (SPEED,
         UPPERS, WHIZZ, SULPHATE, BILLY) even if it was a
         long time ago?

         1   Yes
         2   No
         3   Never heard of it
         4   Don't want to answer

DRQ2A   Have you EVER taken CANNABIS (MARIJUANA,
         DOPE, POT, BLACK, GRASS, HASH, GANJA, BLOW,
         SPLIFFS, JOINTS, DRAW) even if it was a long time
         ago?

         1   Yes
         2   No
         3   Never heard of it
         4   Don't want to answer

DRQ3A   Have you EVER taken COCAINE (COKE, CHARLIE)
         even if it was a long time ago?

         1   Yes
         2   No
         3   Never heard of it
         4   Don't want to answer

DRQ4A   Have you EVER taken CRACK (ROCK, SAND, STONE,
         PEBBLES) even if it was a long time ago?

         1   Yes
         2   No
         3   Never heard of it
         4   Don't want to answer

DRQ5A   Have you EVER taken ECSTASY ('E', DENIS THE
         MENACE) even if it was a long time ago?

         1   Yes
         2   No
         3   Never heard of it
         4   Don't want to answer

DRQ6A   Have you EVER taken HEROIN (SMACK, MORPHINE,
         SKAG, 'H') even if it was a long time ago?

         1   Yes
         2   No
         3   Never heard of it
         4   Don't want to answer

DRQ7A   Have you EVER taken LSD (ACID, TABS, TRIPS)
         even if it was a long time ago?

         1   Yes
         2   No
         3   Never heard of it
         4   Don't want to answer

DRQ8A   Have you EVER taken MAGIC MUSHROOMS (PSI
         LOCYBIN) even if it was a long time ago?

         1   Yes
         2   No
         3   Never heard of it
         4   Don't want to answer

DRQ9A   Have you EVER taken METHADONE (PHYSEPTONE)
         (not prescribed by a doctor) even if it was a long time
         ago?

         1   Yes
         2   No
         3   Never heard of it
         4   Don't want to answer

DRQ12A   Have you EVER taken AMYL NITRATE (POPPERS,
         NITRATES) even if it was a long time ago?

         1   Yes
         2   No
         3   Never heard of it
         4   Don't want to answer

DRQ13A   Have you EVER taken ANABOLIC STEROIDS
         (STEROIDS) **NOT PRESCRIBED A DOCTOR** even if
         it was a long time ago?

         1   Yes
         2   No
         3   Never heard of it
         4   Don't want to answer

DRQ11A   Have you EVER taken TRANQUILLIZERS (eg
         TEMAZEPAM, (JELLIES) VALIUM) **NOT PRESCRIBED
         BY A DOCTOR** even if it was a long time   ago?

         1   Yes
         2   No
         3   Never heard of it
         4   Don't want to answer

DRQ14A   Have you EVER taken GLUES OR SOLVENTS (eg
         LIGHTER FUEL, PETROL, GAS, TIPP-EX) (to sniff or
         inhale)?

         1   Yes
         2   No
         3   Never heard of it
         4   Don't want to answer

DRQ17A   Apart from anything else you have already mentioned,
         have you EVER taken ANYTHING ELSE THAT YOU
         THOUGHT WAS A DRUG **NOT PRESCRIBED BY A
         DOCTOR** but didn't know what it was?

         1   Yes
         2   No
         3   Don't want to answer

Ask if respondent has ever taken amphetamines

DRQ1B   In the last 12 MONTHS have you taken AMPHETA-
         MINES (SPEED, UPPERS, WHIZZ, SULPHATE,
         BILLY) ?

         1   Yes
         2   No
         3   Don't want to answer

Ask if respondent has ever taken cannabis

DRQ2B   In the last 12 MONTHS have you taken CANNABIS (MARIJUANA, DOPE, POT BLACK, GRASS, HASH, GANJA, BLOW, SPLIFFS, JOINTS, DRAW) ?

    1 Yes
    2 No
    3 Don't want to answer

Ask if respondent has ever taken cocaine

DRQ3B   In the last 12 MONTHS have you taken COCAINE (COKE, CHARLIE)?

    1 Yes
    2 No
    3 Don't want to answer

Ask if respondent has ever taken crack

DRQ4B   In the last 12 MONTHS have you taken CRACK (ROCK, SAND, STONE, PEBBLES)?

    1 Yes
    2 No
    3 Don't want to answer

Ask if respondent has ever taken ecstasy

DRQ5B   In the last 12 MONTHS have you taken ECSTASY ('E', DENIS THE MENACE)?

    1 Yes
    2 No
    3 Don't want to answer

Ask if respondent has ever taken heroin

DRQ6B   In the last 12 MONTHS have you taken HEROIN (SMACK, MORPHINE, SKAG, 'H')?

    1 Yes
    2 No
    3 Don't want to answer

Ask if respondent has ever taken LSD

DRQ7B   In the last 12 MONTHS have you taken LSD (ACID, TABS, TRIPS)?

    1 Yes
    2 No
    3 Don't want to answer

Ask if respondent has ever taken magic mushrooms

DRQ8B   In the last 12 MONTHS have you taken MAGIC MUSH-ROOMS (PSILOCYBIN)?

    1 Yes
    2 No
    3 Don't want to answer

Ask if respondent has ever taken methadone

DRQ9B   In the last 12 MONTHS have you taken METHADONE (PHYSEPTONE) (not prescribed by a doctor)?

    1 Yes
    2 No
    3 Don't want to answer

Ask if respondent has ever taken amyl poppers

DRQ12B   In the last 12 MONTHS have you taken AMYL NITRATE (POPPERS, NITRATES)?

    1 Yes
    2 No
    3 Don't want to answer

Ask if respondent has ever taken anabolic steroids

DRQ13B   In the last 12 MONTHS have you taken ANABOLIC STEROIDS (STEROIDS) **NOT PRESCRIBED BY A DOCTOR?**

    1 Yes
    2 No
    3 Don't want to answer

Ask if respondent has ever taken tranquillisers

DRQ11B   In the last 12 MONTHS have you taken TRANQUIL-LIZERS (eg TEMAZEPAM, (JELLIES) VALIUM) **NOT PRESCRIBED BY A DOCTOR**?

    1 Yes
    2 No
    3 Don't want to answer

Ask if respondent has ever taken glues or solvents

DRQ14B   In the last 12 MONTHS have you taken GLUES OR SOLVENTS (eg LIGHTER FUEL, PETROL, GAS, TIPP-EX) (to sniff or inhale)?

    1 Yes
    2 No
    3 Don't want to answer

Ask if respondent has ever taken anything else

DRQ17B   Apart from anything else you have already mentioned, in the last 12 months have you taken ANYTHING ELSE THAT YOU THOUGHT WAS A DRUG (not prescribed by a doctor) but didn't know what it was?

    1 Yes
    2 No
    3 Don't want to answer

Ask if respondent has taken amphetamines in the last 12 months

DRQ1C   In the LAST MONTH have you taken AMPHETA-MINES (SPEED, UPPERS, WHIZZ, SULPHATE, BILLY) ?

    1 Yes
    2 No
    3 Don't want to answer

Ask if respondent has taken cannabis in the last 12 months

DRQ2C   In the LAST MONTH have you taken CANNABIS (MARIJUANA, DOPE, POT, BLACK, GRASS, HASH, GANJA, BLOW, SPLIFFS, JOINTS, DRAW)?

1   Yes
2   No
3   Don't want to answer

Ask if respondent has taken cocaine in the last 12 months

DRQ3C   In the LAST MONTH have you taken COCAINE (COKE, CHARLIE)?

1   Yes
2   No
3   Don't want to answer

Ask if respondent has taken crack in the last 12 months

DRQ4C   In the LAST MONTH have you taken CRACK (ROCK, SAND, STONE, PEBBLES)?

1   Yes
2   No
3   Don't want to answer

Ask if respondent has taken ecstasy in the last 12 months

DRQ5C   In the LAST MONTH have you taken ECSTASY ('E', DENIS THE MENACE)?

1   Yes
2   No
3   Don't want to answer

Ask if respondent has taken heroin in the last 12 months

DRQ6C   In the LAST MONTH have you taken HEROIN (SMACK, MORPHINE, SKAG, H')?

1   Yes
2   No
3   Don't want to answer

Ask if respondent has taken LSD in the last 12 months

DRQ7C   In the LAST MONTH have you taken LSD (ACID, TABS, TRIPS)?

1   Yes
2   No
3   Don't want to answer

Ask if respondent has taken magic mushrooms in the last 12 months

DRQ8C   In the LAST MONTH have you taken MAGIC MUSH-ROOMS (PSILOCYBIN)?

1   Yes
2   No
3   Don't want to answer

Ask if respondent has taken methadone in the last 12 months

DRQ9C   In the LAST MONTH have you taken METHADONE (PHYSEPTONE) (not prescribed by a doctor)?

1   Yes
2   No
3   Don't want to answer

Ask if respondent has taken amyl nitrate in the last 12 months

DRQ12C   In the LAST MONTH have you taken AMYL NITRATE (POPPERS, NITRATES)?

1   Yes
2   No
3   Don't want to answer

Ask if respondent has taken anabolic steroids in the last 12 months

DRQ13C   In the LAST MONTH have you taken ANABOLIC STEROIDS (STEROIDS) **NOT PRESCRIBED BY A DOCTOR?**

1   Yes
2   No
3   Don't want to answer

Ask if respondent has taken tranquillisers in the last 12 months

DRQ11C   In the LAST MONTH have you taken TRANQUILLIZERS (eg TEMAZEPAM, (JELLIES) VALIUM) **NOT PRE-SCRIBED BY A DOCTOR**?

1   Yes
2   No
3   Don't want to answer

Ask if respondent has taken glue or solvents in the last 12 months

DRQ14C   In the LAST MONTH have you taken GLUES OR SOLVENTS (eg LIGHTER FUEL, PETROL, GAS, TIPP-EX) (to sniff or inhale)?

1   Yes
2   No
3   Don't want to answer

Ask if respondent has taken anything else in the last 12 months

DRQ17c   Apart from anything else you have already mentioned, in the LAST MONTH have you taken ANYTHING ELSE THAT YOU THOUGHT WAS A DRUG (not prescribed by a doctor) but didn't know what it was?

1   Yes
2   No
3   Don't want to answer

Ask if respondent has ever taken a drug, but not in the last year

DrugAge   How old were you when you last used any of these drugs?
ENTER YOUR AGE, THEN PRESS THE RED BUTTON

1..97

Ask if informant has used cannabis in last month

Canaw2   You said you have used cannabis, do you ever smoke it mixed with tobacco?

　　　　1　Yes
　　　　2　No
　　　　3　Never smoked cannabis
　　　　4　Don't want to answer

Ask if informant has used two or more drugs in last 12 months

TwoDrgw2   Have you ever used two or more drugs in combination, IN ONE SESSION IN THE LAST 12 MONTHS?

　　　　1　Yes
　　　　2　No
　　　　3　Don't want to answer

Ask if informant has used one or more drugs in last 12 months

DrgAlcw2   Have you ever used one or more drugs in combination with alcohol, IN ONE SESSION IN THE LAST 12 MONTHS?

　　　　1　Yes
　　　　2　No
　　　　3　Don't want to answer

Ask all those aged under 55

DWrong   Please read the following statements and say whether you agree or disagree with them.
　　　　All use of drugs is wrong unless with a doctor's prescription or bought from a chemist.

　　　　1　Strongly agree
　　　　2　Agree
　　　　3　Neither agree nor disagree
　　　　4　Disagree
　　　　5　Strongly disagree

NMind   I don't mind **other** people using drugs.

　　　　1　Strongly agree
　　　　2　Agree
　　　　3　Neither agree nor disagree
　　　　4　Disagree
　　　　5　Strongly disagree

DSafe   Which **one** of the following statements do you agree with?

　　　　1　All drugs are safe to use (as long as you know what you're doing
　　　　2　Some drugs are safe to use (as long as you know what you're doing)
　　　　3　No drugs are safe to use
　　　　4　I don't know whether drugs are safe to use or not

DFriends   Do you know people who use drugs?

　　　　1　Yes
　　　　2　No
　　　　3　Don't know
　　　　4　Don't want to answer

Ask those who have used one or more drugs in the last month

LikeStop   Which one of the following statements best describes you?

　　　　1　I'd like to stop using drugs altogether
　　　　2　I see no need to stop using drugs at the moment
　　　　3　I don't see the need to ever stop using drugs

Ask if LikeStop = would like to stop using drugs

DrugSt1   Which of these statements best describes you?

　　　　1　I intend to stop using drugs within the next month
　　　　2　I intend to stop using drugs within the next six months
　　　　3　I intend to stop using drugs within the next year
　　　　4　I intend to stop using drugs, but not in the next year
　　　　5　I'm unlikely ever to stop using drugs

Ask if LikeStop = sees no need to stop using drugs at the moment

DrugSt2   Which of these statements best describes you?

　　　　1　I'm unlikely ever to stop using drugs
　　　　2　I intend to stop using drugs in the next six months
　　　　2　I intend to stop using drugs within the next year
　　　　3　I intend to stop using drugs, but not in the next year

SEXUAL HEALTH

Ask if aged 16-55 and Nonresp = accepted self-completion or accepted self-completion for sexual health only or completed by interviewer

SexInt   The following questions are about sexual behaviour.
　　　　THE ANSWERS YOU GIVE ARE COMPLETELY CONFIDENTIAL.

　　　　PRESS ENTER TO CONTINUE

W2Sexpar   Have you ever had sexual intercourse?
　　　　Don't forget to include your husband/wife/partner

　　　　1　Yes
　　　　2　No
　　　　3　Don't want to answer

If W2Sexpar = Yes

Tpart   Which one of the following statements applies to you?

　　　　1　I have only had sex with (the opposite sex)
　　　　2　I have had sex with both men and women
　　　　3　I have only had sex with (the same sex)

FirstSex   How old were you on the first occasion that you had sexual intercourse?
　　　　PLEASE TYPE IN THE NUMBER

　　　　10..55

Numparts   Now I would like you to think about the last 12 months, that is since (today's date) 1996. How many sexual partners, in total, have you had intercourse with during that time?
Don't forget to include your husband/wife/partner
PRESS 0 (THE BLUE BUTTON) IF YOU HAVE NOT HAD ANY SEXUAL PARTNERS IN THE LAST 12 MONTHS TYPE IN THE NUMBER THEN PRESS THE RED BUTTON

Ask if Numparts = One

Newpart   Did you have sexual intercourse with this person for the **first** time in the last 12 months?
PRESS 1 FOR YES, PRESS 2 FOR NO THEN PRESS THE RED BUTTON

1   Yes
2   No
3   Don't want to answer

Ask if Numparts = Two or more

Newpart2   Have you had a new sexual partner within the last 12 months?
Please include any partner, even if you only had sexual intercourse on one occasion.

1   Yes
2   No
3   Don't want to answer

Ask if Newpart = Yes or Newpart2 = Yes

Condnew   Now we would like to think of the last occasion that you **first** had sexual intercourse with **someone new**.
Which of the following, if any, were used?
PRESS THE NUMBER OF ALL OF THE ANSWERS THAT APPLY, THEN PRESS THE RED BUTTON

Male condom\sheath\durex
Female condom
The contraceptive pill
Emergency ('morning after') contraception
Other method of protection, including sterilisation
None of these
Can't remember

Ask if used a male or female condom

Whycon   Why did you use a condom on that occasion?
PRESS THE NUMBER OF ALL OF THE ANSWERS THAT APPLY, THEN PRESS THE RED BUTTON

1   For contraception
2   For protection against HIV (the AIDS virus)
3   For protection against other sexually transmitted diseases
4   Other reason
5   Can't remember/Don't know

Ask all respondents

IntrAids   The next two questions are about the risks of getting HIV (the AIDS virus) and other sexually tranmitted diseases.
PRESS THE RED BUTTON TO CONTINUE

AidsRisk   On the whole the risk of someone like me getting HIV (the AIDS) virus is ..

1   very high
2   quite high
3   low
4   or is there no risk at all?
5   Don't know

Stdrisk   On the whole the risk of someone like me getting another sexually transmitted disease (STD) is ..

1   very high
2   quite high
3   low
4   or is there no risk at all?
5   Don't know

CondIntr   Please say how much you agree with the following two statements about using condoms. To go to the first statement, PRESS 1 for YES and PRESS THE RED BUTTON.

Embarass   I would find it difficult to raise the subject of using a condom with a new partner.

1   Strongly agree
2   Agree
3   Neither agree nor disagree
4   Disagree
5   Strongly disagree

Newcond   If in the near future you did have sex with someone new do you think you would ...

1   always use a condom
2   it would depend
3   never use a condom
4   or wouldn't you contemplate having sex?

ThankYou   That is the end of the self-completion. Thank you for your help. All the answers you have given are confidential
To finish the interview, PRESS 1 for YES and PRESS THE RED BUTTON.

Laptop   Now hand the computer back to the interviewer.

ReCtct   If we want to contact you about any future survey, will it be all right if we call on you again?
REMEMBER TO ASK FOR A CONTACT NAME AND NUMBER IN CASE INFORMANT MOVES AND ENTER ON THE YELLOW CARD

1   Yes (unconditional)
2   No (unconditional)
3   Yes (in certain circumstances)

Ask if yes or conditional at Rectct

NumChck   INTERVIEWER CHECK THAT THE TELEPHONE NUMBER YOU HAVE IS CORRECT. IF NOT PLEASE ENTER THE CORRECT TELEPHONE NUMBER ON THE YELLOW CARD

Ask if no at Rectct

RecRef   Code main reason(s) for refusal to the follow-up question.:

    1   Not interested,
    2   Taken too much time,
    3   Have done it once/once is enough,
    4   Questions are too repetitive,
    5   Current survey is too intrusive, objected to
        subject matter

Ask if yes or conditional at Rectct

RecCond   Code main condition(s) to the follow-up:

    1   Contact household beforehand
    2   Only at a convenient time
    3   Someone else (e.g. carer) needs to be there
    4   Don't want to answer questions on financial
        matters
    5   Don't want to answer other types of question

XDontOth   Specify the other types of question informant doesn't
        want to answer:

Ask if yes or conditional at Rectct

LikMov   May I just check, are you likely to be moving from this
        address in the near future?:

    1   Yes
    2   No

Ask if yes at LikMov

MovChck   INTERVIEWER ENTER THE ADDRESS THE
        INFORMANT WILL BE MOVING TO ON THE
        YELLOW CARD

Finish   INTERVIEWER NOW PRESS CTRL + ENTER AND
        THEN CHOOSE 'EXIT VIA ADMIN' TO FILL IN THE
        ADMIN DETAILS OR TO RETURN TO THE MAIN
        MENU

List of figures

Chapter 1   **Page**

1.1   Life events in the last 12 months by sex   5

Chapter 2

2.1   Cigarette smoking status in 1996 and 1997   9

2.2   Odds of trying to give up smoking in the   12
          last 12 months

Chapter 3

3.1   Changes in alcohol consumption between   16
          1996 and 1997 for men and women

3.2   Percentage of respondents whose reported   16
          alcohol consumption was within three units
          of that reported in 1996 by alcohol
          consumption level in 1997 and sex

3.3   Odds of having decreased drinking by more   18
          than 3 units a week between 1996 and 1997

3.4   Odds of having increased drinking by more   19
          than 3 units a week between 1996 and 1997

3.5   Percentage reporting having used a drug in   20
          the past year in 1997 by whether used any
          drug in the past year in 1996 and age

Chapter 4

4.1   Odds of increasing frequency of participation   28
          in sports and exercise activity by more than
          once a week between 1996 and 1997

4.2   Odds of increasing frequency of walking by   29
          more than once a week between
          1996 and 1997

4.3   Odds of increasing participation in home   29
          activities by more than once a week between
          1996 and 1997.

Chapter 5

5.1   Reported changes to diet in the last year by   32
          age and sex

5.2   Odds of an individual changing their diet in   33
          the last year

5.3   Reasons for changing diet in last year   35

List of tables

Chapter 1   **Page**

1.1   Characteristics of the sample by sex   37

1.2   Life events in the 12 months before interview   38
by age and sex

1.3   Percentage reporting two or more life events   39
in the 12 months before interview by selected
characteristics

1.4   Life events in the 12 months before interview   39
by economic activity status

Chapter 2

2.1   Cigarette smoking status and consumption in   40
1996 and 1997 by sex

2.2   Cigarette smoking status in 1997 by cigarette   40
smoking status in 1996 and sex

2.3   Cigarette smoking status in 1996 and 1997 by   41
age and sex

2.4   Reported changes in daily cigarette   41
consumption between 1996 and 1997 by
cigarette smoking status in 1996 and sex

2.5   Perceived changes in cigarette consumption   42
in the last year by cigarette smoking status
in 1996

2.6   Perceived changes in cigarette consumption   42
in the last year by reported changes in
consumption

2.7   Number of attempts to give up smoking and   43
whether has tried to cut down on smoking in
the last 12 months by whether wanted to give
up and when intended to give up in 1996 and
sex

2.8   Number of attempts to give up smoking and   44
whether has tried to cut down on smoking in
the last 12 months by whether had ever tried
to give up and how easy smokers thought it
would be to go without a cigarette for a day

Chapter 3

3.1   Alcohol consumption level (AC rating) and   45
mean weekly number of units by year and sex

3.2   Alcohol consumption level in 1997 by   45
alcohol consumption level in 1996 and sex

3.3   Change in alcohol consumption between   46
1996 and 1997 by sex

3.4   Change in alcohol consumption between   46
1996 and 1997 by age and sex

3.5   Change in alcohol consumption between   47
1996 and 1997 by consumption in 1996
and sex

3.6   Change in alcohol consumption between   47
1996 and 1997 by respondent's attitude to
his/her drinking in 1996 and sex

3.7   Perceived changes in drinking in the last year   48
by age and sex

3.8   Perceived changes in drinking in the last year   48
by alcohol consumption in 1996

3.9   Perceived change in drinking by change in   48
alcohol consumption between 1996 and
1997 and sex

3.10   Main reason for drinking more than a year   49
ago by sex

3.11   Main reason for drinking less than a year   49
ago by sex

3.12   Percentage who had used drugs in the past   49
year by drug category, year and sex

3.13   Drug usage in 1996 by type of usage in 1997   50
and age

3.14   Change in drug use between 1996 and 1997   50
by respondent's attitude to his/her drug use
in 1996

3.15   Category of drugs used by change in overall   51
use between 1996 and 1997

3.16   Change in cannabis use between 1996 and   51
1997

Chapter 4

4.1   Frequency of participation in activity by   52
year and sex

4.2   Frequency of participation in different types   52
of at least moderate intensity activity for 30
minutes or more by sex in 1996 and 1997

4.3   Frequency of at least moderate intensity   53
activity for 30 minutes or more in 1997 by
frequency in 1996 and sex

4.4   Change in activity group between 1996 and   53
1997 by age and sex

4.5   Changes in frequency of activity group in   54
1996 by age and sex

4.6   Frequency of at least moderate intensity   55
activity for 30 minutes or more in 1997 by
frequency in 1996, type of activity and sex

		Page
4.7	Percentage of men and women who increased their participation in different types of activity by overall changes in physical activity group	55
4.8	Change in activity group between 1996 and 1997 by whether, in 1996, respondent would like more and when they intended to take more exercise by sex	56
4.9	Change in frequency of different types of activity between 1996 and 1997 by whether, in 1996, respondent would like more exercise and when they intended to take more exercise by sex	57
4.10	Perceived change in activity comparing 1997 with a year ago by age and sex	58
4.11	Perceived change in activity comparing 1997 with a year ago by change in reported activity and sex	58

Chapter 5

5.1	Changes to diet in the last year by age and sex	59
5.2	Changes to diet in the last year by social class based on own current or last job, and sex	60
5.3	Changes to diet by 1996 intentions to change diet	61
5.4	Reasons for changing diet in the last year by age	61

Section 6

6.1	Age at first intercourse by age and sex	62
6.2	Number of sexual partners in the last 12 months by year and sex	63
6.3	Number of sexual partners in the last 12 months in 1997 by number of sexual partners in the last 12 months in 1996 and sex	63
6.4	Number of sexual partners in the last 12 months in 1997 by assessment of risk of getting HIV (the AIDS virus) in 1996 and sex	64
6.5	Number of sexual partners in the last 12 months in 1997 by assessment of risk of getting another sexually transmitted disease in 1996 and sex	64
6.6	Respondents' assessment of the likelihood of 'someone like me getting HIV (the AIDS virus)' by year and sex	65
6.7	Respondents' assessment of the likelihood of 'someone like me getting another sexually transmitted disease' by year and sex	65

		Page
6.8	Whether would find it difficult to raise the subject of using a condom with a new partner by year and sex	65
6.9	Whether would use a condom if 'in the near future they did have sex with a new partner' by year and sex	65
6.10	Whether reported a new partner in the last 12 months in 1997 by whether reported a new partner in the last 12 months in 1996 and sex	66
6.11	Percentage using a condom with a new partner by year and sex	66

Section 7

7.1	Number of occasions of sunburn in the last 12 months by year and sex	67
7.2	Occasions on which respondents use suncream by year and sex	67
7.3	Whether having a suntan is important by year and sex	68
7.4	Number of occasions of sunburn in the last 12 months in 1996 and 1997 by sex	68
7.5	Number of occasions of sunburn in the last 12 months in 1997 by whether used a suncream in 1996 and sex	69
7.6	Number of occasions of sunburn in the last 12 months in 1997 by whether a suntan was important in 1996 and sex	70
7.7	Number of occasions of sunburn in the last 12 months in 1997 by whether agreed having a suntan is attractive in 1996 and sex	71
7.8	Number of occasions of sunburn in the last 12 months in 1997 by whether agreed having a suntan makes me feel healthier in 1996 and sex	72

Appendix A

A.1	The sample of respondents from the 1996 survey	78
A.2	Response of adults to follow-up interview	78
A.3	Response of adults aged 16-55 to the self-completion module	78
A.4	Distribution of responders to 1996 HEMS compared to Labour Force Survey (LFS) estimates for England by age and sex	79
A.5	Distribution of responders to 1996 HEMS compared to Labour Force Survey (LFS) estimates for England by standard region	79

		Page
A.6	Distribution of responders to 1996 HEMS compared to GHS 1994 by marital status	80
A.7	Distribution of responders to 1996 HEMS compared to Labour Force Survey by ethnic origin and sex	80
A.8	1996 age-sex-region weights	81
A.9	Characteristics of responders and non-responders to the 1997 survey	82
A.10	Selected estimates for responders and non-responders to the 1997 survey	83
A.11	1997 weighting classes	84
A.12	Standard errors and 95% confidence intervals for socio-demographic variables	85
A.13	Standard errors and 95% confidence intervals for general health variables	86
A.14	Standard errors and 95% confidence intervals for smoking variables	86
A.15	Standard errors and 95% confidence intervals for drinking variables	87
A.16	Standard errors and 95% confidence intervals for drugs variables	88
A.17	Standard errors and 95% confidence intervals for physical activity variables.	89
A.18	Standard errors and 95% confidence intervals for nutrition variables	90
A.19	Standard errors and 95% confidence intervals for sexual health variables	91
A.20	Standard errors and 95% confidence intervals for behaviour in the sun variables	91